INTERMITTENT FASTING PLAN

step by step guide on how to loss weight using the 16:8 method with intermittent fasting plan

by David Carol

4

BOOK 1

BOOK 2

INTERMITTENT FASTING

DIET PLAN

The complete and flexible diet plan to lose weight through intermittent fasting

By David Carol

Respective authors own all copyrights not held by the publisher.

The information herein is offered for informational purposes solely and is universal as such. The presentation of the information is without a contract or any guarantee assurance. The trademarks used are without any consent, and the publication of the trademark is without permission or backing by the trademark owner. All trademarks and brands within this book are for clarifying purposes only and are owned by the owners themselves s, not affiliated with this document.

Chapter 1. Intermittent Fasting and Cholesterol

How might you bring down cholesterol without meds? What's more, what befalls your cholesterol in the event that you do intermittent fasting?

Elevated cholesterol is viewed as a treatable danger factor for cardiovascular infection, for example, coronary episodes and strokes. There are numerous subtleties to cholesterol which I would prefer not to get into, yet generally, the fundamental division has been between Low Density Lipoprotein (LDL) or 'terrible' cholesterol, and High Density Lipoprotein (HDL) or 'great' cholesterol. All out cholesterol gives us minimal valuable data.

We additionally measure fatty substances, a kind of fat found in the blood. Fat is put away in fat cells as fatty oils, yet in addition skims around unreservedly in the body. For instance, during fasting, fatty substances get separated into free unsaturated fats and glycerol. Those free unsaturated fats are utilized for energy by a large portion of the body. So fatty substances are a type of put away energy. Cholesterol isn't. This substance is utilized in cell fix (in cell dividers) and furthermore utilized for to make certain chemicals.

14

The Framingham Heart investigations of the mid 1960s set up that high blood cholesterol levels just as high fatty oils are related with coronary illness. This affiliation is a lot more fragile than the vast majority envision, however results were somewhat improved when LDL was considered independently from HDL. Since cholesterol is found at the site of athermanous plaques, the blockages in the heart, it appeared to be natural that high blood levels assumes a part in 'obstructing the supply routes'.

The inquiry, consequently, became, what causes high blood levels of cholesterol? The originally thought was that high dietary admission of cholesterol would prompt high blood levels. This was disproven many years prior. One may (erroneously) imagine that diminishing dietary cholesterol may decrease blood cholesterol levels. Notwithstanding, 80% of the cholesterol in our blood is created by the liver, so diminishing dietary cholesterol is very fruitless. Studies show that how much cholesterol we eat has next to no to do with how much cholesterol is in the blood. Whatever else he got off-base, he got this correct eating cholesterol doesn't raise blood cholesterol. Each and every examination done since the 1960s has shown this reality over and over. Eating more cholesterol doesn't raise blood levels.

In any case, it has taken far longer for this data to arrive at the general population. Dietary Guidelines for Americans, distributed like clockwork, has more than once focused on bringing down dietary cholesterol as though it had an effect. It doesn't. Anyway, if dietary cholesterol didn't raise blood cholesterol, what did?

1.1 Low Fat Diets and Cholesterol

The following idea was that bringing down dietary fat, particularly immersed fats, and may help lower cholesterol. While false, there are as yet numerous who trust it. In the 1960's the Framingham Diet Study was set up to explicitly search for an association between dietary fat and cholesterol. This was a similar Framingham as the acclaimed Heart Studies, however references to the Framingham Diet study are for all intents and purposes non-existent. All things considered, the discoveries of this examination showed no connection between dietary fat and cholesterol at all. Since these outcomes conflicted with the common 'astuteness' of the time, they were smothered and never distributed in a diary. Results were classified and taken care of in a dusty corner.

However, different examinations all through the following not many years tracked down a similar adverse outcome. The Tecumseh study contrasted blood cholesterol levels with dietary fat and cholesterol. Regardless of whether blood levels were high, medium or low, each gathering essentially ate a similar measure of fat, creature fats, soaked fats and cholesterol. Dietary admission of fat and cholesterol doesn't impact blood cholesterol much.

WHAT IS
CHOLESTEROL?

Cholesterol is mainly comprised of fat
and lipoproteins. A lipoprotein is comprised of
cholesterol, protein, and fat (triglycerides).

In certain examinations, amazingly low-fat eating regimens can bring down the LDL (awful cholesterol) somewhat, yet they additionally will in general lower the HDL (great cholesterol) so it is questionable whether by and large wellbeing is improved. Different examinations show no such bringing down. For instance, here's an investigation in 1995, where 50 subjects were taken care of either a 22% or a 39% fat eating regimen. Standard cholesterol was 173 mg/dl. Following 50 days of a low fat eating routine, it dove to 173 mg/dl. Goodness. High-fat weight control plans don't raise cholesterol much by the same token. Following 50 days of high fat weight control plans, cholesterol expanded barely to 177 mg/dl.

A great many individuals attempt a low-fat or low-cholesterol diet without understanding that these have effectively been demonstrated to fizzle. I hear this constantly. At whatever point someone is told their cholesterol is high, they say "I don't comprehend. I've removed every single greasy food". Indeed, decreasing dietary fat won't change your cholesterol. We've known this for quite a while. There are minor changes, best case scenario. Anyway, what to do? Statins, I presume?

A little starvation can truly support the normal debilitated man than can the best drugs and the best specialists. Studies show that fasting is a basic dietary procedure that can fundamentally bring down cholesterol levels.

Presently, there are numerous contentions about lipids that I don't wish to get entanglement in. For instance, there are numerous insights concerning molecule size and computations of all out molecule numbers and more current particles and so on that are past the extent of this conversation. I will restrict this conversation to the exemplary HDL/LDL/and fatty oils.

1.2 High Density Lipoprotein

'Great' cholesterol (HDL) is defensive, so the lower the HDL, the higher the danger of CV infection. This affiliation is in reality significantly more remarkable than that for LDL, so we should begin here. These are affiliations just, and HDL is essentially a marker for illness. Medications that raise HDL don't ensure against coronary illness, similarly as not make you more youthful.

Quite a while prior, Pfizer emptied billions of dollars into investigating a medication (a CETP inhibitor). This medication been able to fundamentally expand HDL levels. On the off chance that low HDL caused coronary failures, this medication could save lives. Pfizer was so secure with itself, it burned through billions of dollars attempting to demonstrate the medication compelling.

The examinations were finished. What's more, the outcomes were stunning. Stunningly awful, that is. The medication expanded passing rate by 25%. Indeed, it was murdering individuals left and right like Ted Bundy. A few additional medications of a similar class were tried and had a similar executing impact. Only one more outline of the 'Connection isn't Causation' truth.

All things considered, we care about HDL since it is a marker of illness, similarly as a fever is frequently the apparent indication of a basic contamination. Assuming HDL is diminished, it very well might be a sign that the basic circumstance is likewise declining. What befalls HDL during fasting? You can see from the diagram that 70 days of substitute day by day fasting had a negligible effect upon HDL levels. There was some reduction in HDL however it was negligible.

The narrative of fatty oils (TG) is comparative. TGs are markers of sickness, yet they don't cause it. Niacin is a medication that builds HDL and lower TG without especially impact on the LDL.

Study tried whether niacin would have any cardiovascular advantages. The outcomes were shocking. Incredibly terrible, that is. While they didn't execute individuals, they didn't help them all things considered. Furthermore, there were parcels part results. In this way, TG, similar to HDL is just a marker not a causer of infection.

What befalls TG during fasting? There's an immense 30% reduction in TG levels (great) during substitute every day fasting. Truth be told, fatty oil levels are very delicate to slim down. Yet, it isn't diminishing dietary fat or cholesterol that makes a difference. All things considered, decreasing carbs is by all accounts the principle factor that lessens TG levels.

1.3 Triglycerides

The LDL story is considerably more combative. The statin drugs lower LDL cholesterol effectively, and furthermore diminishes CV illness in high danger patients. Yet, these medications have different impacts, frequently called the pleiotropic (influencing various frameworks) impacts. For instance, statins likewise diminish aggravation, as demonstrated by the decrease in incendiary marker. Anyway, is it the cholesterol bringing down or the pleiotropic impacts that are answerable for the advantages?

This is a decent inquiry to which I don't have an answer yet. The best approach to advise is lower LDL utilizing another medication and check whether there are comparable CV advantages. The medication preliminary likewise had some CV advantages, yet they were very feeble. To be reasonable, the LDL bringing down was additionally very humble.

Another class of medications has the ability to decrease LDL a ton. The inquiry, however is whether there will be any CV advantage. Early signs are very certain. Be that as it may, it is a long way from authoritative. So the chance exists that LDL may assume a causal part here. This is, all things considered, why specialists stress such a huge amount over holding LDL down.

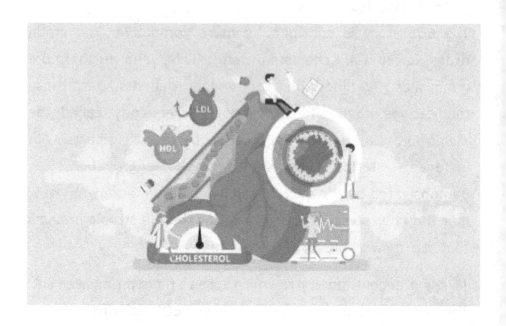

What befalls LDL levels during fasting? Indeed, they go down. A ton. Preposterous long stretches of substitute day by day fasting, there was about a 25% decrease in LDL (generally excellent). Undoubtedly, medications can diminish them about half or more, however this basic dietary measure has practically a large portion of the force of quite possibly the most remarkable classes of drugs being used today.

In mix with the decrease in body weight, safeguarded sans fat mass, and diminished midsection outline, unmistakably fasting produces some incredible enhancements in these cardiovascular danger factors. Remember to include the diminished LDL, decreased fatty oils and protected HDL.

Be that as it may, for what reason does fasting work where ordinary weight control plans fall flat? Basically, during fasting, the body changes from consuming sugar to consuming fat for energy. Free unsaturated fats (FFA) are oxidized for energy and FFA combination is decreased (body is consuming fat and not making it). The lessening in triacylglycerol amalgamation brings about an abatement in VLDL (Very Low Density Lipoprotein) discharge from the liver which brings about brought down LDL.

The best approach to bring down LDL is to cause your body to consume it off. The slip-up of the low-fat eating routine is this taking care of your body sugar rather than fat doesn't cause the body to consume fat it just causes it to consume sugar.

1.4 Low Density Lipoprotein
The LDL story is substantially more petulant. The statin drugs lower LDL cholesterol capably, and furthermore decreases CV infection in high danger patients. Be that as it may, these medications have different impacts, frequently called the pleiotropic (influencing numerous frameworks) impacts. For instance, statins additionally lessen aggravation, as demonstrated by the decrease in a fiery marker. Things being what they are, is it the cholesterol bringing down or the pleiotropic impacts that are liable for the advantages?

This is a decent inquiry to which I don't have an answer yet. The best approach to advise is lower LDL utilizing another medication and check whether there are comparable CV advantages. The medication in the preliminary likewise had some CV advantages, yet they were incredibly powerless. To be reasonable, the LDL bringing down was likewise very humble.

New class of medications called the PCSK9 Inhibitors has the ability to lessen LDL a ton. The inquiry, however is whether there will be any CV advantage. Early signs are very certain. However, it is a long way from complete. So the chance exists that LDL may assume a causal part here. This is, all things considered, why specialists stress such a great amount over holding LDL down.

What befalls LDL levels during fasting? All things considered, they go down. A ton. Ridiculous long stretches of substitute every day fasting, there was about a 25% decrease in LDL (excellent). Certainly, medications can decrease them about half or more, yet this straightforward dietary measure has practically a large portion of the force of perhaps the most remarkable classes of meds being used today.

In blend with the decrease in body weight, protected sans fat mass, and diminished midriff outline, obviously fasting produces some incredible upgrades in these cardiovascular danger factors. Remember to include the decreased LDL, diminished fatty substances and protected HDL.

However, for what reason does fasting work where normal weight control plans fizzle? Basically, during fasting, the body changes from consuming sugar to consuming fat for energy. Free unsaturated fats (FFA) are oxidized for energy and FFA amalgamation is diminished (body is consuming fat and not making it). The lessening in triacylglycerol blend brings about a reduction in VLDL (Very Low Density Lipoprotein) emission from the liver which brings about brought down LDL.

The best approach to bring down LDL is to cause your body to consume it off. The slip-up of the low-fat eating routine is this taking care of your body sugar rather than fat doesn't cause the body to consume fat it just causes it to consume sugar. The error of the Low-Carb, High-Fat eating routine is this giving your body heaps of fat causes it to consume fat, yet it will consume what's coming into the framework (dietary fat). It will not haul the fat out of the body.

Here's the reality for those 10,000 foot view, spare me the subtleties sort of people. Fasting has the accompanying impacts:

- Decreases weight
- Keeps up lean mass
- Diminishes midsection size
- Insignificant change in HDL
- Sensational decreases in TG
- Sensational decreases in LDL

That is all acceptable. Regardless of whether this will all convert into improved heart results, I don't have the response for you. My theory is yes. Be that as it may, fasting consistently reduces to this. There are altogether these advantages. There's next to no danger. What do you need to lose (other than a couple of pounds)? For individuals stressed over cardiovascular failures and strokes, the inquiry isn't "The reason would you say you are fasting?", yet "For what reason would you say you are not fasting?"

1.5 How to Control Cholesterol by Intermittent Fasting Diet Plan

The impetus for intermittent fasting's medical advantages, they say, is metabolic exchanging, which happens when cells change from utilizing glucose for energy to utilizing ketone bodies, and afterward back once more.

A commonplace carb rich eating routine of three dinners per day in addition to snacks gives a sizable amount of glucose to influence cells. Yet, during fasting, glucose runs out and the liver reacts by changing unsaturated fats over to ketone bodies, an interaction known as ketosis. Ketone bodies give consistent, fat-inferred energy and seem to direct proteins and atoms identified with wellbeing and maturing, they compose.

Spotlights on two explicit systems: the two-days seven days fasting plan rehearsed and the time-limited timetable rehearsed by another specialist, which requires burning-through the day's food in a window of six to eight hours and fasting the remainder of the time. Studies have not yet thought about the overall adequacy of the two regimens.

Both eating plans advocate a restorative eating regimen, yet do exclude directions about what food sources to eat or the number of calories to devour. In the event that somebody's typical eating regimen is unfortunate and they change to intermittent fasting it will likely profit their wellbeing.

Specialist started shortening the time period in which he eats in 1982, he said, when he surrendered breakfast since it upset his stomach prior to bicycling to his doctoral level college grounds. He presently devours his day's calories somewhere in the range of 1 and 7 p.m., eating generally vegetables, organic products, nuts, entire grains, beans and yogurt.

Likewise started contemplating intermittent fasting during the 1990s as a feature of his examination into Alzheimer's and other neurodegenerative infections. "We realized each and every other day fasting had an enemy of maturing impact on rodents as in it expanded life expectancy, so we inquired as to whether this adjustment of eating example would secure nerve cells and keep them working better more," he says. "We found that it did."

Exploration on the possible advantages of intermittent fasting is as yet in its beginning phases. One test is getting study members to stay with the prohibitive eating plans. In their paper, by limiting eating only one day a week or eating in a 10-hour window.

Dawson concurs that the routine requires discipline, particularly in the initial not many weeks. He makes it much more testing by putting his two low-calorie days close to one another, generally Sunday to Monday or Monday to Tuesday. What you're attempting to do is push your body to a ketotic state. On the off chance that you do it a subsequent day, the whole second day you're in a ketotic state, and I think you get more advantage.

The low-calorie days can trigger headaches yet it is normally ready to forestall them by drinking a great deal of water. Before the second's over day, it is covetous. The mind is revealing to me it needs energy. In any case, I'm as yet ready to work at a beautiful undeniable level. I feel somewhat sharper, somewhat crisper. It's likely whatever the ketotic state has incited my body to deliver.

1.6 Intermittent Fasting Helps Improve your Heart Health

Possibly. Scientists aren't sure why, yet it appears to be that some sort of fasting seriously limiting food and drink for a specific timeframe can conceivably improve some danger factors identified with heart wellbeing.

There are an assortment of mainstream ways to deal with fasting, including substitute day fasting and time-confined eating. Substitute day fasting includes eating ordinarily one day and fasting or eating minimal the following. Time limitations include eating just between specific hours of the day, for example, between 11 a.m. furthermore, 7 p.m.

It's hard to determine what impact ordinary fasting has on your heart wellbeing on the grounds that numerous individuals who regularly quick do as such for wellbeing or strict reasons. These individuals for the most part watch out for not smoke, which additionally can diminish coronary illness hazard. In any case, a few examinations have shown that individuals who follow a fasting diet may have preferred heart wellbeing over individuals who don't quickly.

Normal fasting and better heart wellbeing may likewise be connected to the manner in which your body uses cholesterol and sugar. Customary fasting can diminish your low-thickness lipoprotein, or "terrible," cholesterol. It's additionally believed that fasting can improve the manner in which your body processes sugar. This can lessen your danger of putting on weight and creating diabetes, which are both danger factors for coronary illness.

Nonetheless, there are worries about the possible symptoms of normal fasting for specific individuals or in explicit conditions. Fasting isn't suggested for:

- Individuals with dietary problems and the individuals who are underweight
- Ladies who are pregnant or breastfeeding
- Individuals taking diabetes meds
- Individuals with end-stage liver illness

The impacts of fasting on heart wellbeing look encouraging, yet more examination is expected to decide if standard fasting can diminish your danger of coronary illness. In case you're thinking about customary fasting, converse with your primary care physician about the advantages and disadvantages. Remember that a heart-solid eating regimen and practicing routinely additionally can improve your heart wellbeing.

Chapter 2. Impact of Intermittent Fasting on the Profile of Lipid

Intermittent fasting, whose reported benefits include improved lipid profiles and weight loss, has gotten a lot of press in the scientific and popular press. This survey aims to bring together findings from studies that looked at people's lipid profiles after a period of intermittent fasting using an itemized audit, as well as suggestions for a physiological instrument that takes into account eating habits and weight loss. Intermittent fasting, both normal and hypo caloric, can be a dietary technique for improving lipid profiles in healthy, overweight, and dyslipidemia people by lowering absolute cholesterol, LDL, and HDL, fatty compounds, as well as an increase in HDL levels. Nonetheless, the majority of studies that look into the effects of intermittent fasting on lipid profiles and body weight loss are observational and based on Ramadan fasting, which necessitates a large sample size and precise diet details. Randomized clinical preliminaries with a bigger example size are expected to assess the intermittent fasting impacts essentially in patients with dyslipidemia.

Sub-ideal HDL is a prognostic marker of cardiovascular sickness. South Asia has a high predominance of problematic HDL contrasted with different pieces of the world. Intermittent fasting (IF) is a kind of energy limitation which may improve serum HDL and different lipids along these lines diminishing

31

the danger of cardiovascular sicknesses. The point of the investigation was to assess the impact of IF on lipid profile and HDL-cholesterol in an example of South Asian grown-ups.

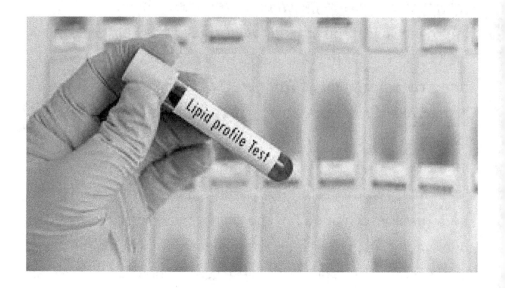

2.1 Introduction

Human fasting is considered as food forbearance and even drinks between 4 h to three weeks. Viable utilization of human fasting includes the pre-logical period of a few research center testing, preoperative and postoperative which disproved with admission is essential, as gastrointestinal injury. Intermittent fasting (IF) is a limited taking care of period begins in strict and profound practices. The most examined kind of intermittent fasting IF happens in the sacred month of Ramadan, which is a period that millions of Muslims avoid caloric and water admission from dawn to nightfall. By and large, the Ramadan day is The Ramadan day is divided into two parts: fasting and non-fasting. .

Different kinds of intermittent fasting are likewise considered, for example, substitute day fasting e.g., 1 day or more seven days fasting and intermittent fasting with a more extended fasting period during the day, for instance, 16 h of fasting for 8 h of non-fasting. These sorts of intermittent fasting don't need limitation of water consumption since they have no association with religion. Intermittent fasting has acquired great and well known repercussion, being presented as a taking care of strategy under specific conditions in the clinical practice. Studies that intricate pathways made based on the creature examinations may prompt overestimation of intermittent fasting in regards to biochemical markers, for example, the customary profile of lipid including high-thickness lipoprotein (HDL), low-thickness lipoprotein (LDL), complete cholesterol and fatty oils. Intermittent fasting can be viewed as a low energy convention that prompts profile of lipid improve by low few energy or potentially body weight decrease. Henceforth, the caloric admission and weight reduction assessments are critical to explore the organic impacts of intermittent fasting on profile of lipid. This audit meant to unite considers that dissected the impacts of intermittent fasting IF on profile of lipid in people, accentuating the physiological systems.

2.2 Foundation of Intermittent Fasting Diet Plan

It is very much recorded that dyslipidemia, portrayed by high grouping of serum complete cholesterol (TC), low-thickness lipoprotein cholesterol (LDL-C) and fatty oils (TG) with low degrees of high-thickness lipoprotein cholesterol (HDL-C), is connected to cardiovascular infection (CVD). A few investigations have shown that low HDL-C, with ordinary LDL-C and fatty oil levels can be as hazardous for coronary wellbeing as high LDL-C. HDL-C inverts cholesterol transport and lessens the atherosclerotic weight. HDL-C likewise has mitigating, hostile to oxidative, against thrombotic, hostile to apoptotic, and vasodilator properties. Different elective ways for overseeing dyslipidemia incorporate way of life change, ordinary exercise and moderate liquor utilization.

Intermittent fasting (IF) can be embraced as a way of life alteration for great wellbeing and adjusted lipid profile. In the event that is kind of energy limited taking care of convention known since long from strict and social foundations. On the off chance that has been widely concentrated in creature models. Such investigations demonstrate that IF improves lipid profile, shields the heart from ischemic injury, and constricts post-MI cardiovascular renovating. Different logical examinations have been directed on people to distinguish the job of various IF strategies including substitute day fasting, caloric limitation, Ramadan fasting and occasional fasting and so forth Substitute day fasting (ADF) diminishes body weight by 3–7% more than 2–multi month, and improves lipid profiles and pulse. It was proposed that fasting decidedly impacts metabolic biomarkers and cardiovascular wellbeing while long haul impacts ought to be investigated. A clinical preliminary of ADF in grown-ups with corpulence discovered it as a viable strategy for weight decrease and decrease in coronary conduit illness hazards. Furthermore, one clinical preliminary discovered ADF successful for weight decrease in individuals with typical and overweight. Mix of substitute day fasting with actual work reports more noteworthy changes in body arrangement and plasma lipid profile and diminishes cardiovascular danger when contrasted with singular medicines. It is tracked down that intermittent fasting IF is as powerful for weight the executives as ceaseless calorie limitation for about two months. The diminished caloric admission and weight reduction may clarify the impacts of IF on the lipid profile which might be meant enhancements in cardio metabolic wellbeing.

Ramadan fasting considers have shown blended impacts on wellbeing. A few investigations discovered decrease in body weight while others report negligible change. Comparative intermittentities are accounted for the lipid profile and blood glucose levels too. One clarification could be the frustrating factors like the fasting length, drugs, dietary propensities, social standards and actual work. Different components may incorporate methodological contrasts, occasional changes, geological area, sunshine openings and so forth

The current examination preliminary was intended to explore the impacts of intermittent fasting IF on lipid profile in grown-ups. It was speculated that intermittent fasting IF will improve the lipid profile and may forestall cardiovascular illnesses. The examination convention was not the same as other recently considered intermittent fasting IF techniques as it required day time 12 h fasting for 3 days per week for about a month and a half. It had likeness with Ramadan fasting in that the quick was kept from dawn to nightfall however it was unique in relation to Ramadan fasting in the viewpoint that Ramadan fasting requires every day fasting for four consistent weeks. In this examination, intermittent fasting IF was characterized as fasting for 3 days in seven days for about a month and a half.

2.3 Intermittent Fating Methods

A point by point writing research in English was conveyed so as to distinguish great investigations and to portray and merge observational and mediation information that gave boundaries of the profile of lipid through people, like HDL, VLDL, LDL, absolute cholesterol and fatty oils. In equal, body weight and dietary data were likewise considered as information. To improve the confirmations in regards to organic help contemplates that pre-owned more point by point markers than the conventional profile of lipid were additionally investigated, consequently proposing physiological instruments to explain the improvement of the profile of lipid through intermittent fasting.

A 6-week semi trial (non-randomized) clinical preliminary was directed on members with low HDL. Members of the benchmark group were prescribed not to change their eating regimen. The mediation bunch was prescribed too quickly for 12 h during day time, three times each week for about a month and a half. Heartbeat rate, pulse, body weight, midsection periphery, serum lipid profile, and blood glucose levels were estimated at pattern and following a month and a half.

This was a semi exploratory clinical investigation. Individuals were educated through messages, calls and individual contacts. The Good Clinical Practice rules was followed. Subsequent to disclosing the investigation convention to the members, composed educated assent was gathered. Members didn't get any motivator, financial or something else, for taking part in this investigation. Test size was determined by investigating the past intermittent fasting preliminary example sizes. The force of the examination for huge improvement in HDL cholesterol was 80%, with an importance level of 5%.

Consideration rules included age of 20–70 years, with serum HDL 40 mg/dl for men and 50 mg/dl for ladies. Pregnant ladies and people with self-announced cardiovascular infections or some other co-dismalness were prohibited. Screening was performed and lipid profile was directed to affirm HDL levels.

A sum of 40 subjects (20 in each gathering) were selected the examination.

2.4 Can Intermittent Fasting Affect the Lipid in Humans?

Intermittent fasting (IF) is a limited taking care of period arose out of strict and otherworldly customs. The most contemplated kind of intermittent fasting happens in the sacred month of Ramadan. Meanwhile, a huge number of Muslims stop food varieties and refreshments utilization from dawn to nightfall. In general, Ramadan day comprise in 12 h fasting and 12 h taking care of. Other than Ramadan, different kinds of intermittent fasting IF are likewise examined. Substitute day fasting is an expansive term so have a few statements. At some point or two spans days seven days fasting are most expanded models. The presence of caloric admission in the fasting day is questionable. A few examinations consider unhealthy limitation as a fasting day, for instance, 25% ingestion of all out caloric use in one day, and caloric overcompensation consumption on one more day for example non-fasting day. An interest day by day kind of intermittent fasting IF is 16 h fasting for 8 h taking care of, be that as it may, there can be every day types with seriously fasting span, as 16 to 20 h fasting for 4 to 8 h taking care of. These kinds of intermittent fasting don't need limitation of water admission since they have no association with religion. Weight reduction techniques are great for profile of lipid improvement. There is a great connection among heftiness and dyslipidemia over supportive of inclination from fat tissue.

The pathophysiology of the regular dyslipidemia saw in corpulence is multifactorial, in which overconsumption of calories is vital. Low-calorie diets can upgrade the profile of lipid; similarly, intermittent fasting can prompts profile of lipid improve by low energy and additionally body weight decrease. Lipid improvement through intermittent fasting IF can happen with or without changes in weight reduction. Observational examinations dependent on Ramadan are the larger part, without a doubt showing numerous limits, for example, the absence of food review from calories to macronutrients. Contrasting the pre and post intermittent fasting period, HDL levels can increment somewhere in the range of 1 and 14 mg/dL, LDL levels decline somewhere in the range of 1 and 47 mg/dL, all out cholesterol levels decline somewhere in the range of 5 and 88 mg/dL and fatty substances levels decline somewhere in the range of 3 and 64 mg/dL. Although observational examinations are most of intermittent fasting IF research, there are randomized clinical preliminaries showing upgraded profile of lipid relationship with weight reduction by goodness of intermittent fasting IF program. It is tried two kinds of substitute day fasting: 1) High-fat, Low-Carb diet; 2) Low-fat, High-Carb diet. They showed diminished cholesterol, LDL fatty oils and cholesterol, levels and bodyweight in the two gatherings. Late examination by likewise tried High-fat, Low-Carb diet and Low-fat, High-Carb diet over substitute day fasting with more prominent development, comparing to a half year. Conversely it is found simply adlibbing HDL levels, while didn't diminish LDL, fatty oils and cholesterol levels. Moro et al. discovered lipid improvement solid opposition prepared guys during two months of norm caloric intermittent fasting. There was expanded HDL and diminished LDL levels in the intermittent fasting bunch, while ordinary eating routine gathering didn't change

2.5 Intermittent Fasting Proposed Mechanisms

The increment of tumor corruption factor alpha and a few cytokines are related with deteriorating of the profile of lipid. In the investigation interleukin (IL) - 2 and IL-8 and TNF-a levels were diminished after the time of Ramadan in eutrophic and fat, in any case, IL-1 and IL-6 levels weren't diminished. Despite the fact that there was a lessening in the serum fatty oil, the more powerless to blood vessel entrance. Taking everything into account, the instruments that legitimize the improvement of the profile of lipid through intermittent fasting are to be expected. Likely the instrument of intermittent fasting IF for the improvement of lipoproteins, cholesterol and serum fatty oils are like the works of art that happen through fat mass misfortune. Most importantly, dietary quality ought to be thought of. The sort of standard caloric or hypo caloric intermittent fasting improves lipoproteins by more prominent unsaturated fat oxidation and regulation of Apo lipoproteins. In the liver, the oxidation of unsaturated fats is expanded through higher articulation of peroxisome proliferator-actuated receptor alpha and peroxisome proliferator-initiated receptor-gamma co activator 1-alpha in the fasting state.

Through increment of unsaturated fat oxidation in the liver, the aggregation of fatty substances in the hepatocytes diminishes, in this manner diminishing the creation of low thickness lipoprotein (VLDL). Through diminishing the VLDL creation consequently decreasing degrees of VLDL and TG in the circulation system, since makes VLDL, serum Apo B levels are likewise decreased. Through lessening these variables that include VLDL, thusly the LDL and sdLDL are likewise diminished. In equal, serum Apo B levels are likewise decreased, for Apo B is important for LDL just as sdLDL and VLDL. Intermittent fasting may likewise diminish the declaration of cholesteryl ester move protein (CETP) when related with fat mass misfortune. The CETP is a protein liable for moving cholesterol esters from HDL to VLDL, being answerable for bringing down HDL levels and expanding VLDL levels. Accordingly, the diminishing in CETP through fasting can be another reality that can build HDL. Innate in the improvement of serum cholesterol, the plausible instrument of fasting and cholesterol decrease happens through enzymatic activity. Fasting diminishes the declaration of sterol administrative component restricting protein, reducing the activity of a few compounds answerable for cholesterol amalgamation.

2.6 Analysis of Weight Loss

With respect to dietary admission and weight reduction, when looking at the pre and post intermittent fasting time frames, eleven examinations had a great decline in the body weight, which changed between1.1 and 6.5 kg. Mediations brought about a more noteworthy abatement of body weight, as the examinations, both happening during 2 and a half year, separately. Inside the gatherings that broke down the progressions of the fat mass after the intermittent fasting, six of them showed measurable greatness in the diminishing when contrasted with the pattern. Two examinations that showed a decline in the fat mass after Ramadan discovered a decrease of 1 kg and 3.6 kg, though the biggest diminishing of fat mass was confirmed in the gathering.

2.7 Analysis of Cardiovascular Outcome

Examination of cardiovascular infection results is foremost for a superior appraisal of the profile of lipid through intermittent fasting. To this end, from a complete 448 patients in an examination that assessed the cardiovascular danger potential, 122 patients occasionally rehearsed strict fasting, and there was a 54% decrease in the danger of coronary conduit illness in subjects who followed the intermittent fasting, a worth got after multivariate change for age, sex, weight file, dyslipidemia, diabetes, smoking, and family ancestry. Then again, in a new cross-sectional investigation with an enormous example, the non-breakfast people had a higher danger of atherosclerosis contrasted with the individuals who ingested fatty for breakfast (20% of day by day calorie admission). Nonetheless, non-breakfast patients, when contrasted with the high caloric admission gathering of his supper, shown ominous boundaries, for example, higher level of focal stoutness, body weight, weight file, abdomen periphery, dyslipidemia and glycaemia; they were more seasoned, with a higher level of ladies and smokers; ingested all the more day by day calories, creature protein, complete fat, cholesterol, handled food sources and cocktail; and, they ate less dietary vegetables and entire grains. In seeing this, it is hurried to say that food hardship at breakfast prompts cardiovascular occasions.

2.8 Data Collection and Intervention of Intermittent Fasting

The representatives who consented to take an interest in the preliminary were called for screening. They were approached to bring their lipid profile result from the most recent a month, if accessible. The people without such past lipid profile reports were approached to come after 10–12 h of fasting so a lipid profile test could be performed. People with low HDL levels showed either by the past reports or by presently performed screening lipid profiles were taken a crack at the examination. Screening and enrolment were finished in 3 a month. At that point selected members were welcome to an assigned room in the Multidisciplinary research facility where polls with respect to members' eating standard and actual work of

43

member were finished. Body weight, midriff perimeter, tallness and circulatory strain were estimated. Muscle to fat ratio and water content were estimated by an impedance scale. Blood was gathered for lipid profile testing and glucose assessment. Members were called again following a month and a half whereby a similar body boundaries were estimated and fasting blood was gathered.

The members were appropriated into two gatherings as indicated by their gathering inclination; Control and Intervention. Educated assent structure was endorsed by every one of the members. Intercession bunch was encouraged too quickly for 12 h during day time for just 3 days/week for about a month and a half. The mediation bunch was told to take their normal eating routine in the non-fasting period. The benchmark group proceeded with their typical dietary example and were encouraged to roll out no improvements in way of life. Consistence was checked through calls and messages each week for about a month and a half. In spite of the fact that there are no detailed antagonistic impacts of intermittent fasting, the contact number of a specialist was given to members in the event of any crisis or concern.

2.9 Strong Points and Limitations

Audits that feature intermittent fasting as a compelling technique for profile of lipid control have not made express the worth of profile of lipid markers and dietary information. To stay away from incomprehension and improve the understanding of this audit: we normalized all units of the profile of lipid in mg/dL through traditional conditions, investigated the deficiency of body weight and taking care of previously and not long after the intermittent fasting time frame; since it is an agreement that weight reduction, low calorie and the variance of the lipid profile is influenced by both genetics and dietary consistency.

Besides, it is an agreement that ladies show a more great status than men chiefly the HDL and this survey give the appraisal of the lipid of the two sexes through intermittent fasting can improve the lipid in people yet is important to think about the term, sex and weight reduction. Taken together, this survey remembered these contemplations for request to give better awareness of physiological varieties. Significantly, one certainty to be considered is the utilization of prescriptions, particularly lipid-bringing down drugs. Most of studies chose in this audit didn't utilize drugs and most subjects were sound. Just intermittent fasting in patients who were utilizing the lipid-bringing down drug, like statins, since the patients were dyslipidemia. Didn't search improvement in the lipid in the two people accordingly it is hurried to consider intermittent fasting as the principle technique for the dyslipidemia control this ought not be viewed as a treatment to substitute the utilization of lipid-bringing down drugs. Dissecting the lipid after intermittent fasting follow-up is fundamental to comprehend the repercussion of this dietary technique in the lipid supportive of documents. Of the couple of studies that proved the lipid following multi month of the intermittent fasting time frame expanded HDL levels continued as before following multi month of the Ramadan fasting by examines. A restriction of this survey isn't to have reached a systematization for the incorporation of research articles.

2.10 Analysis of Intermittent Fasting Data

Information are introduced as mean standard deviation. Nonetheless, information is introduced as mean contrast standard mistake mean. The degree of importance was set for all performed two-sided tests. To distinguish changes over the long haul and separate contrasts between the gatherings, a rehashed measures with factors time (pre, post) into gathering of intermittent fasting (IF, Control) was performed to test for communication impacts. On account of huge collaboration impacts, t-tests were determined for any pre to post contrasts. For metabolic danger factors, information have been changed with mean of body weight of the whole example at pattern.

2.11 Result

An aggregate of 40 members were taken on the examination (20 in each gathering), while 35 (20 control and 15 mediation) finished the preliminary and were remembered for information investigation of the investigation. Body estimations, including body weight, BMI and midriff circuit, showed huge connection impacts, demonstrating that there were bigger decreases in the intermittent fasting IF bunch than in the benchmark group. Critical connection impacts were additionally noticed for aggregate, HDL, and LDL cholesterol with bigger enhancements in the intermittent fasting IF bunch.

Out of 70 people, 40 satisfied the consideration standards and were selected the investigation – 20 in each gathering. 35 members (87.5%) finished the examination. Five dropouts from the intercession bunch were because of individual reasons or failure to agree with the fasting system.

The gauge portrayal of members including age, sexual orientation, pulse, BMI level and subtleties of their current ailment. The itemized survey with respect to eating schedules and active work at benchmark level and after post examination showed no distinction, every one of the members followed their equivalent day by day schedules as prompted.

The progressions in boundaries at benchmark and post a month and a half report. Body estimations including body weight and BMI showed huge collaboration impacts and time impacts while midriff circuit showed critical association impact as it were. Critical association impacts were shown by HDL, complete cholesterol and LDL with non-huge time impacts. Moreover, muscle versus fat, fatty substances and blood glucose didn't show any critical cooperation impacts.

The mean changes in body estimations, lipids, and blood glucose levels from standard to post-treatment for the control and mediation gatherings and the aftereffects of post-hoc examinations of inside bunch change. The IF bunch had critical decreases in body weight, BMI and abdomen outline. The mean contrasts for intermittent fasting IF bunch were additionally huge for all out cholesterol), HDL, LDL and fatty oils. There were no critical changes for any of the boundaries for the benchmark group. Notwithstanding, it ought to be noticed that the between-bunch distinction in change didn't arrive at measurable importance for fatty oils.

The correlation of changes in body estimations, lipid and blood glucose levels of control and mediation bunches at gauge and post intercession with importance level of connection impact.

2.12 Hence Intermittent Fasting Helps in Lowering Lipids

The investigation recommends that IF has the capability of improving the lipid profile and lessening body weight and abdomen boundary. These outcomes are in accordance with different examinations showing that various sorts of intermittent fasting IF, including Ramadan fasting and elective day fasting, decrease body weight and lipid levels. Studies joining IF with actual work and looking at changed sorts of intermittent fasting IF likewise recommend that intermittent fasting IF can be a viable way of life alteration for lessening the dangers of cardiovascular illnesses. In any case, the greater part of the intermittent fasting IF clinical preliminaries in the writing were led for brief timeframes and huge scope randomized controlled preliminaries with longer length and subsequent meet-ups are not accessible. Long haul studies ought to be led to approve their adequacy and wellbeing.

Incorporated information from various preliminaries and reasoned that various sorts of intermittent fasting IF can build HDL, decline LDL, decline TC and diminishing TG. When contrasted with different kinds of intermittent fasting IF, our technique seems protected, viable and can be embraced in everyday life, with no extra monetary or actual weight. People can consolidate intermittent fasting IF into their ways of life without stressing over any additional endeavors to get ready low calorie dinners. The 12-h quick may be kept up by an early breakfast and eating at a fitting time, which works for non-weekend days and ends of the week. Nonetheless, it very well may be hard for individuals working late evenings or having a functioning public activity with incessant eating out schedules. This was likewise seen in the current examination; 5 individuals exited from the investigation because of their chaotic and occupied timetable and couldn't keep up fasting period for multi day/week.

Recently led preliminaries have referenced that intermittent fasting of 12–36 h brings about a metabolic change prompting a separate of fatty substances into unsaturated fats and glycerol and transformation of unsaturated fats to ketone bodies in the liver. During fasting, unsaturated fats and ketone bodies give energy to cells and tissues. Studies recommended that particle regulation in the liver prompts articulation that builds unsaturated fat oxidation and its creation prompting expanded HDL levels, though different reductions which causes diminished hepatic fatty substances and LDL levels.

The principle constraints of this examination included non-randomization of the investigation populace. Moderate to extreme dyslipidemia patients were excluded from the investigation. Other significant impediment was the exit five members from the mediation gathering of the examination which may have expanded the size of the outcomes. It was a solitary focused and limited scope study lacking information on food admission and record of caloric admission.

Chapter 3. Trimming your Waistline by Intermittent Fasting Diet Plans

Intermittent fasting, in which people quick occasionally, is an inexorably famous weight reduction routine. To comprehend the momentary impacts of such a routine, we present an instance of intermittent fasting with information assortment that emulates the single-case plan.

A sound however somewhat overweight grown-up male went through complete quick for two entire days and continued with ordinary eating for five days, and rehashed the cycle multiple times. Information were gathered from three periods: standard (multi week); fasting (three weeks); post-fasting (multi week). Estimations taken every day incorporate weight, muscle versus fat proportion, temperature, pulse, blood glucose, just as midsection and hip circuits. Blood tests were directed week by week for wellbeing screening and to get perceptions on lipid profile, high-touchy C-receptive protein, hemoglobin A1C (HbA1c), and uric corrosive.

The member lost 1.3 kilograms (kg) in body weight. Muscle versus fat proportion didn't contrast a lot. Fasting caused an intense drop in the blood glucose level, which was reestablished after continuing ordinary eating. Complete cholesterol dropped definitely following the main fasting cycle however bounced back 15% higher than benchmark prior to dropping down. Fasting likewise incidentally raised uric corrosive levels, circulatory strain, and internal heat level. HbA1c and abdomen and hip outlines were not influenced by fasting. Improvement in provocative marker was noticed.

This case shows that intermittent fasting can initiate transient weight reduction and lessen intense provocative marker in a sound grown-up, however not muscle versus fat proportion and lipid profile. Comparative single-contextual analysis configuration can be applied across a training based organization for between case replication.

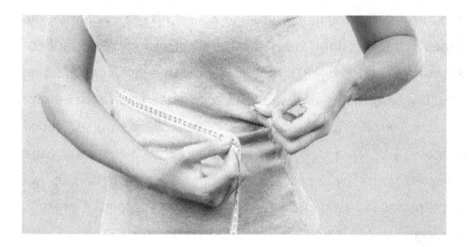

3.1 Introduction

Intermittent fasting is an enveloping term covering any eating plan that shifts back and forth among fasting and non-fasting periods. The various sorts of intermittent fasting incorporate total substitute day fasting, altered fasting regimens, and time-confined taking care of. Intermittent fasting has become a very well-known dietary arrangement and a way of life approach for weight reduction. Of course, intermittent fasting has been broadly advanced on the regular, computerized, and online media with wellbeing cases, for example, working with weight and muscle versus fat misfortune, bringing down the dangers of type II diabetes and cardiovascular infections, advancing cell recovery, diminishing and oxidative pressure, and just as easing back the maturing cycle.

These cases are undoubtedly upheld by a huge assemblage of examination on creatures and a few human mediation concentrates with promising researches. A new audit of the metabolic impacts of intermittent fasting discovered proof that upholds the act of intermittent fasting to initiate supported upgrades in human wellbeing. A deliberate survey distributed in 2018 discovered intermittent fasting to be successful in decreasing weight independent of weight list. Besides, great diminishes in fat mass, low-thickness lipoproteins, and fatty substances were reliably detailed in completely included examinations. In any case, this precise survey included just four great clinical preliminaries. A 2018 meta-investigation of six clinical preliminaries likewise discovered intermittent fasting to be more successful than no treatment for weight reduction except for not better than persistent energy limitation.

While proof is arising to help the important impacts of intermittent fasting as a non-pharmacological way to deal with improve wellbeing, there is still a lot of obscure as to the effectiveness of different types of intermittent fasting, the replicable of the metabolic impacts found in creature studies to people, and the drawn out security of energy limitation. Moreover, there is as yet the test of making an interpretation of examination proof into training with no settled clinical rules set up.

With the expanding ubiquity of intermittent fasting, clinicians, particularly those in essential consideration, will definitely look with patients who are intrigued by the overeager cases on the media and wish to evaluate intermittent fasting. Rather than excusing it as a craze and hazard having the patients go through intermittent fasting unaided, a clinician can examine with the patient on the accessible proof and any potential wellbeing suggestion. Given that administered fasting is protected and with simply gentle to direct and known responses, should the patient endure, the clinician can consider working with the patient to contemplate the time course, changeability, and impact of the mediation in clinical practice, if time and cost license. Thusly, clinicians can acquire further experiences to customize weight the board techniques for the patient and to relieve any potential wellbeing hazard.

3.2 Case Presentation of Intermittence Fasting Diet Plan

A solid however imperceptibly overweight Asian male (age 48 years) was intrigued to investigate the utilization of intermittent fasting as a way of life approach for weight reduction. He was 83 kilograms (kg) beforehand and had effectively diminished his weight to 61 kg by embracing an exacting plant-based eating routine and exercise over a time of three years. He was respectably dynamic and strolled for in any event an hour every day with his pedometer check averaging 12,500 stages in the course of recent years. He was not determined to have any ongoing conditions. He didn't have any set of experiences of gastrointestinal issues other than a disengaged episode of draining duodenal ulcer when he was a teen, which had since been settled after treatment with ranitidine.

Notwithstanding proceeding to keep a plant-based eating regimen and a moderate exercise, he was encountering steady weight gain to 66 kg in the course of the most recent two years. With a stature of 1.64 meters (m), his weight list was 24.53 kg/m2, returning him to the overweight classification under the World Health Organization's corpulence rules for Asia-Pacific populaces. His midsection outline was 88.5 cm, just marginally underneath the stomach corpulence remove point for Asians (90 cm in men). With a family background of stroke, he was quick to decrease his weight back to the typical reach.

3.3 Data Collections and Interventions

The case individual decided to seek after a variation of the famous five-two (5:2) intermittent fasting routine (an altered fasting routine with extreme energy limitation for two days of the week and not obligatory eating for the other five days). Rather than devouring 20% to 25% of energy needs on two non-back to back fasting days of the week according to the standard 5:2 convention, the individual selected to notice total fasting with no energy-containing food varieties or refreshments burned-through for two sequential days of the week, making the all-out long periods of fasting being 48 hours or all the more however not more than 60 hours. The individual had experienced 18 hours of fasting as a feature of his strict practice before which gave him certainty that he could continue for two back to back days without food. He additionally planned to keep up his typical active work level all through the fasting periods however much he could.

To evaluate the adequacy of this weight reduction plan and its metabolic impact, the individual agreed to take day by day estimations on weight, muscle versus fat mass and proportion, temperature, pulse, fasting blood glucose, just as midriff and hip boundaries. All estimations were taken utilizing family wellbeing observing hardware after waking prior to devouring any food or beverages. Every day actual work level (estimated in the all-out number of steps) was additionally observed utilizing a pedometer worn during waking hours. The individual likewise consented to go through blood tests week after week at a business clinical research facility for security screening and to acquire perceptions on lipid profile, high-touchy C-responsive protein, hemoglobin A1C (HbA1c), and uric corrosive. During the fasting time frame, blood tests were taken toward the beginning of the day following two successive long stretches of fasting before any dinner.

For wellbeing, the individual was urged to drink sufficient water to stay away from parchedness. He was to notice manifestations including unpredictable heart cadence, perspiring, precariousness, nervousness, abundance yearning, and sickness. To forestall hypoglycemia, he was advised to drink one to two tablespoons of nectar in warm water at regular intervals until the indications died down. Extra blood glucose test ought to be taken to guarantee the blood glucose level didn't drop. He was advised to quit fasting and look for clinical assistance if the indications continued returning and blood glucose kept up at sub level. He could likewise decide to surrender fasting whenever.

Information were gathered more than three times of five weeks (35 days): benchmark (multi week); fasting (three weeks); post-fasting (multi week). The length was dictated by the case individual as he proposed to utilize the fasting routine as a momentary weight support approach. Correlation of the seven-day midpoints of the post-fasting day by day estimations of weight and muscle to fat ratio to the benchmark midpoints was utilized to decide the adequacy of the eating routine arrangement. The individual was likewise encouraged to keep a diary on his abstract insight of fasting.

Body Weight

The time course of the body weight changes. At pattern, the everyday weight estimations range between 65.5 kg to 66.4 kg with a mean of 65.9 kg. A quick drop in weight is recognizable on two successive fasting days and the drop proceeds with one more day with resumption of eating before a bounce back on the ensuing days. After three patterns of intermittent fasting, weight estimations on the post-fasting week settle between a lower scopes of 64.2 kg to 65.1 kg with a mean of 64.6 kg. A decrease of 1.3 kg is noticed, addressing a 2% loss of starting body weight.

Mass and Body Fat Ratio

Dissimilar to changes in the body weight after some time, no unmistakable example rises up out of the visual investigation of muscle versus fat proportion estimations. The benchmark normal of muscle versus fat proportion is 19.1% (Range: 18.6% to 19.5%). In correlation, the post-fasting normal muscle versus fat proportion is 18.8% (Range: 18.2% to 19.4%). This adjustment of muscle versus fat proportion is viewed as too little to even think about being of any clinical importance.

The time course of the progressions in muscle versus fat mass which intently follows the progressions in muscle versus fat proportion. The underlying normal muscle to fat ratio mass is 12.61 kg (range: 12.35 kg to 12.83 kg), and the post-fasting normal of muscle versus fat mass is 12.17 kg (range: 11.83 kg to 12.45 kg). A drop of 0.44 kg, which is about 3.6% of introductory muscle to fat ratio mass, is identified.

Physical Activity

The everyday actual work estimated in the quantity of steps recorded. Albeit the individual expected to keep up his ordinary active work level all through the fasting period, there had all the earmarks of being a drop in actual work levels during fasting days. In any case, we can't determine any reasonable example since there he likewise recorded lower active work levels during a few non-fasting days. Looks at the normal quantities of steps each week more than five periods. Apparently the individual normally decreased his active work levels during fasting periods. Thus, any progressions in body weight and fat can't be a consequence of any expanded active work level.

Blood Glucose

The everyday variances in fasting blood glucose level. Notwithstanding for an apparently descending pattern during the benchmark time frame before the principal fasting week, fasting blood glucose level seems to gleam around 5.0 to 5.8 plant moles per liter. The underlying descending pattern during the gauge, while fascinating, isn't of any clinical importance since such variance is well inside the ordinary reach.

A radical drop in fasting blood glucose levels is seen toward the beginning of each fasting period, particularly during the principal fasting period which measures at 3.4 plant moles per liter. With the resumption of eating, the fasting blood glucose level immediately reestablished to the past non-fasting level. This perception is steady for an ordinary non-diabetic person.

Other Daily Measurements

Estimations of internal heat level with mean of 35.78 degrees Celsius and scope of 35.3 to 36.4 °C, systolic circulatory strain with mean of 101.24 millimeters of mercury (mmHg) and scope of 89 to 111 mmHg, just as diastolic pulse with mean of 60.24 mmHg and scope of 52 to 72 mmHg, taken all through the perception period are well inside the ordinary reaches. Visual examination of the information design over the long run doesn't uncover any impact of fasting on these boundaries. Estimations of the midriff and hip peripheries likewise show no recognizable change.

Lipid Level

The progressions in lipid profile over the long run. A drop in all lipid profile boundaries is seen after the initial two continuous long periods of fasting. Be that as it may, all out cholesterol level seems to bounce back and ascend after ensuing patterns of fasting and arrive at its top at 206 milligrams for each deciliter (mg/dL) multi week after the last two continuous fasting days prior to dropping back to 186 mg/dL, a level higher than 175 mg/dL at gauge. Thus, different patterns of complete 5:2 fasting seem to raise the all-out cholesterol level from the ideal reach to the scope of marginal high (200 and 239 mg/dL).

The variances in absolute cholesterol level are expected fundamentally to the progressions in the low-thickness lipoprotein (LDL) cholesterol and fatty substances. The high-thickness lipoprotein (HDL) cholesterol gives off an impression of being discouraged by fasting, subsequently, the complete cholesterol to HDL proportion ascends after the last two fasting cycles.

Notwithstanding the vacillations in boundaries, the subject's lipid profile stays at the sound level at post-fasting.

High-sensitive Hemoglobin A1c, and Uric acid

The fiery marker is decreased radically from 2.0 milligrams per liter at pattern to 0.6 mg/L after the initial two back to back long stretches of fasting. It drops further in the following two cycles and reliably remains at 0.3 mg/L at post-fasting.

As opposed to it, HbA1c isn't influenced by intermittent fasting as it stays reliably inside the scope of 5.3% to 5.6% all through. This more extended term glycemic control measure stays unaltered by momentary intermittent fasting.

The degree of uric corrosive is another biomarker that is obviously influenced by the act of intermittent fasting. The uric corrosive level ascents from 7.0 mg/dL to over 9.0 mg/dL during the fasting time frames and drops back to 7.0 mg/dL post-fasting. Fasting pushes the serum uric corrosive level past the ordinary reach.

3.5 Subjective Experiences and Adverse Effect

All blood tests show no anomaly or radical change in liver profile and complete blood tally all through three periods.

The case individual detailed no genuine unfriendly occasion and no gastrointestinal grumbling. His fasting diary contained sections of "harder to get into rest than typical" and "interfered with rest" on the second day of fasting and feeling "feeble and mixed up when initially stood up after waking" during the principal fasting cycle. He additionally portrayed the sensation of "gentle snugness at the head likened to the involvement with high elevation". These were side effects of gentle hypoglycemia as his blood glucose level was arriving at a low of 3.4 mill mole per liter. As exhorted, the individual drank one glass of nectar water as a prudent step and the side effects dispersed. He didn't think that it's important to screen his blood glucose level once more. During the following two cycles, these encounters died down as the body "probably become accustomed to it". The experience of "harder to get into rest than ordinary" stayed through the three cycles however.

By and large, the subject was happy with the consequences of intermittent fasting and would consider doing it once more.

3.6 Discussion

We realize next to know about the transient impact of intermittent fasting as a weight support approach on sound non large subjects in the writing. Most intermittent fasting contemplates have study terms of 3 months or more to examine chronicity. Detailed a huge mean deficiency of 2.5 of starting body weight and a critical decrease of the underlying fat mass with a mean of 4.0 of 1% among 16 nonfat members (half male) following 21 days of substitute day fasting with no caloric admission each and every other day. Such discoveries are predictable with our perceptions for this situation with the deficiency of around 2% of beginning body weight and 3.6% of starting fat mass following three weeks of intermittent fasting with no caloric admission on two back to back days out of each week. The weight reduction is little as the individual has effectively lost huge load previously. His metabolic rate has acclimated to his present weight, making it difficult to accomplish intense weight reduction in only 35 days.

Nonetheless, in another perception study, revealed no critical change in mean load of eight sound guys was found subsequent to going through intermittent fasting each second day for 20 hours over a length of 15 days. Essentially, discovered no distinctions in body weight of eight sound subjects in a get over preliminary contrasting substitute day fasting with the standard eating routine more than about fourteen days. Subsequently, we propose that for intermittent fasting to be compelling in accomplishing about 2% of weight reduction in a non-corpulent subject, a base span of three weeks is required. While a 5% decrease in weight is usually thought to be as clinically critical for the counteraction and treatment of stoutness, huge medical advantages are accomplished in relationship with humble (under 3%) weight reduction in grown-ups who embrace and support actual work joined with an energizing eating routine. Consequently, three weeks of intermittent fasting can be another choice for momentary weight support mediation for non-stout people notwithstanding actual exercise and legitimate eating regimen.

Fasting is known to incite intense changes in blood glucose level. It noticed a critical mean decrease in 30 members (66.7% female) following one day of water-just quick and a bounce back of 0.327 mill mole per litter subsequent to eating was continued. For our situation, the example of intense drop and bounce back is also noticed and the blood glucose level keeps up at the lower level on the second day of fasting. It likewise creates the impression that the decrease in blood glucose level isn't as exceptional in the second and third patterns of fasting, implying the capacity of the body to adjust to the fasting condition. Further investigations with more subjects are expected to affirm this glucoregulatory perception. When looking at mean contrast in post-fasting blood glucose level to that of the standard following three weeks of intermittent fasting, we don't discover any distinction for this situation which is predictable with other intermittent fasting investigations of comparative span.

An audit discovered most intermittent fasting examines announced improvement in lipid profile including diminishing complete cholesterol, LDL, fatty substances and expanding HDL levels. Conversely, for our situation, decrease in all lipid profile boundaries seems, by all accounts, to be only an intense response of the body to the effect of the initial two successive long stretches of fasting. Raised degrees of all out cholesterol, LDL, and fatty substances during the last piece of the fasting time frame is distinguished. This can be because of individual fluctuation or the impact of complete 5:2 fasting. Since current proof depends for the most part on the other day fasting or time-confined taking care of (counting Ramadan quick), there is inadequate comprehension on the impact of intermittent fasting on lipid profile with over 24 hours of complete energy limitation. This can be a space of additional exploration.

Weight reduction is known to connect with a decrease in the degree of C-responsive protein (CRP), an aggravation marker ensnared in the danger of creating constant illnesses including cardiovascular infection, diabetes, and malignant growth. Shockingly, the discoveries from intermittent fasting considers were blended in for certain investigations discovered critical enhancements in aggravation markers including CRP while others didn't. In the current case, the progressions in the marker as an impact of intermittent fasting is surprising (from 2.0% to 0.3%). Nonetheless, we ought to decipher this perception with alert and not sum up.

Aggravation marker is an intense stage reactant of the aggravation reaction which is influenced by numerous conditions. It's anything but an action for the danger of irritation. Besides, the body may combine less CRP in fasting because of the absence of protein sources. Consequently, any adjustment of CRP doesn't really address an adjustment of starting clinical state as other provocative cycles may influence the CRP esteems. More examination on the impact of intermittent fasting on aggravation marker is required.

In overweight and stout subjects just as patients with type II diabetes, intermittent fasting was similarly viable in improving longer-term glycemic control pointer estimated by the HbA1c inside a year time span, contrasted with constant energy limitation. Notwithstanding, in investigations of more limited span and in non-diabetic populace, diminished HbA1c has not been reliably illustrated. As HbA1c is mirroring the total glycemic history of the previous a few months, the vacillation in blood glucose level brought about by transient intermittent fasting has no impact on this marker as demonstrated in the current case. Subsequently, HbA1c is certainly not a suitable measure here. The 1, 5-anhydroglucitol test can be a superior marker for present moment glycemic control to examine the impacts.

We notice the ascent of serum uric corrosive during fasting. This is normal. During fasting, the body utilizes different stores for energy which incorporate the breakdown of put away proteins/amino acids and fats. Uric corrosive is a byproduct of this catabolic cycle. Fasting has been accounted for to increment uric corrosive in the writing. Announced the straight increment of serum uric corrosive level with the term of Ramadan quick among 16 volunteers. Runcie and Thomson likewise discovered the event of hyperuricemia in 42 corpulent patients treated with all out fasting. In any case, the impact was clearly innocuous as none of the patients create intense gout.

This case report imitates the single subject examination plan which can be a helpful apparatus by and by based essential consideration research. The tedious pattern of intermittent fasting mentions it characteristic for objective facts to be made with numerous times of standard (for example non-fasting days) and on numerous occasions for mediation (for example fasting days) according to the essential A-B single-subject plan. While perceptions from a solitary case can't be summed up, a similar procedure can be duplicated across a training based organization for additional comprehension of the impacts of intermittent fasting on various subjects.

Assortment of cases can be utilized for meta-examination and inferential

Conclusion

Intermittent Fasting might be a dietary technique to help in the improvement of the lipid in solid, fat and dyslipidemia people, diminishing all out cholesterol, LDL, fatty oils and expanding HDL levels. Nonetheless, most of studies that break down the intermittent fasting IF impacts on the lipid and body weight reduction are observational and need definite data about diet. Randomized clinical preliminaries with a bigger example size are expected to assess the IF impacts essentially inpatients with dyslipidemia.

This case shows that three weeks of intermittent fasting can instigate transient weight and fat mass misfortune with a decrease in intense incendiary marker in a solid grown-up, however not muscle versus fat proportion and lipid profile. Complete fasting for two entire days of the week is all around endured by the person. Despite the fact that improvement in lipid profile through intermittent fasting is ordinarily announced in the writing, this case shows a transitory ascent in lipid profile boundaries during fasting despite the fact that the impact is by all accounts transient. Transient rise of serum uric corrosive level is likewise noticed. Comparative single-subject examination configuration can be applied across a training based organization for between case correlation and investigation.

This examination recommends that intermittent fasting may secure cardiovascular wellbeing by improving the lipid profile and raising the imperfect HDL. Intermittent fasting might be received as a way of life mediation for the counteraction, the executives and treatment of cardiovascular issues.

INTERMITTENT FASTING

DIET PLAN

The Ultimate Guide to Accelerate Weight Loss, Promote Longevity, and Increase Energy with a New Lifestyle

Chapter 1. The Impact of Intermittent Fasting on your Brain

Lately intermittent fasting has become a well-known food pattern and diet. However, aside from simply assisting with weight reduction, it has a lot more medical advantages.

With amusement park only a couple a long time behind us, an exceptional season has started. As per Christian practices, late-winter was a time of fasting, as numerous food varieties were somewhat scant during this season. While the festival of fair remaining parts famous in certain pieces of the Netherlands, the custom of fasting subsequently, initially explicit to meat and liquor, is just maintained by a moderately modest number of individuals. Nonetheless, different kinds of fasting have formed into food patterns as of late. One of those patterns is intermittent fasting (IF). In the event that doesn't just assist with weight reduction, yet additionally decreases the danger of some constant infections (e.g., hypertension, irritation and neurodegenerative sicknesses) and even advantages our cerebrum.

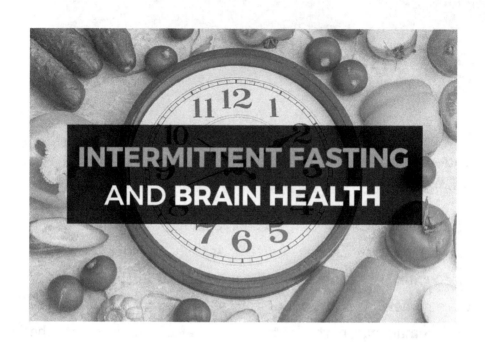

1.1 Introduction

Intermittent Fasting IF isn't such a lot of an eating routine as it is just eating as indicated by a timetable. The time windows in which you are permitted to eat are limited and there are expanded time-frames with practically zero food admission. There are a few group who abandon nourishment for 16 hours consistently and eat just during the leftover eight hours (this is likewise called a period confined eating regimen). Another exceptionally regular eating design is the 5:2 eating regimen, where you eat typically for five days consistently, however eat almost no or nothing on two nonconsecutive days out of each week.

After just around six hours of fasting, the body begins delivering a greater amount of the alleged human development chemical (HGH). This chemical changes digestion to support fat consuming over protein use. Consequently, proteins can generally be utilized for cell fix and the improvement of synapse working. HGH additionally decreases irritation in the body and invigorates up guideline of autophagy. Autophagy is an interaction where there's a tidy up and reusing of unused or harmed cell parts ("cell garbage") and along these lines advances the wellbeing and endurance of our cells. Also, intermittent fasting IF expands the levels of a protein called cerebrum determined neurotropic factor

(BDNF). Together, every one of these cycles have a beneficial outcome on mind working.

1.2 How Intermittent Fasting Influence our Brain?

Every one of these cycles (protein saving, decrease of irritation, autophagy and increment of BDNF creation) advantage our mind. From one viewpoint they lessen the harm to synapses by, for instance, holding down provocative responses and disposing of waste in the cerebrum. Then again, they likewise animate appropriate mind work, by advancing cell fix and adding to the development of new synapses and associations between them, accordingly working with correspondence inside the cerebrum. BDNF specifically adds to this structure cycle, and deficiencies in this protein have been connected to intellectual issues during maturing like dementia. So intermittent fasting IF has a neuroprotective impact and thusly adds to solid maturing.

On the off chance that isn't an eating routine that you can simply begin starting with one day then onto the next. It requires preparing to adapt well to the times of food hardship. Be that as it may, and still, at the end of the day, intermittent fasting IF isn't for everybody. For instance, it ought to be kept away from by individuals who are underweight, in danger of unhealthiness, experiencing a dietary issue or are having issues with keeping up their glucose levels. So before you begin changing your dietary patterns radically, it is consistently a smart thought to counsel a wellbeing proficient.

1.3 Try Intermittent Fasting for Brain Health at Home

Talking about the most recent neuroscience research on intermittent energy limitation (IER). IER, as the name infers, includes intermittently confining energy admission, or calories. You can do this severally. In one strategy you seriously limit calories (think 400-500 absolute admission each day) a few days per week; in another you bind your food admission to a 8-hour time frame each day; and in one more you quick once every week for a 24-to 36-hour duration.

The advantages of intermittent fasting for metabolic wellbeing are as of now truly settled. In non-human creature models just as in people, IER prompts weight reduction and diminished muscle versus fat; brings down pulse and resting pulse; and improves hazard markers for malignancy, diabetes, and cardiovascular infection. This is genuine in any event, when the quick's general calorie utilization is equivalent to a non-quicker (on the grounds that, for instance, the quicker burns-through a bigger number of calories during his non-fasting periods than he would something else). Just by offering yourself an incidental reprieve from eating, at that point, you offer your body a major kindness, regardless of whether you don't eat less generally.

It's turning out to be certain that the upsides of IER are significantly further coming to, with colossal ramifications for cerebrum wellbeing. Human and non-human creature examines have shown that IER increments synaptic pliancy (an organic marker of learning and memory), upgrades execution on memory tests in the older, prompts the development of new neurons, advances recuperation after stroke or horrible mind injury, diminishes hazard for neurodegenerative sicknesses like Alzheimer's and Parkinson's illness, and may improve personal satisfaction and intellectual capacity for those all around determined to have these infections. IER has additionally been appeared to assume a precaution and remedial part in temperament problems like tension and sadness.

The compensations of IER for metabolic and cerebrum wellbeing are interceded by various complex organic components, however the fundamental thought behind the science is straightforward: Periodically challenge your phones and natural frameworks (by food hardship) in a controlled way, and these phones and frameworks will get more grounded, more productive, and better ready to deal with the day by day focuses on that come their direction. It's the very essential thought that underlies weight-preparing and different types of activity. We harm our muscles (a smidgen) to develop them.

Given the expanding logical agreement and the enormous likely result for mind and body wellbeing, I chose in the wake of recording our digital broadcast that I would be wise to put my cash or my vacant fork where my mouth is and check IER out. In spite of the fact that the human IER examines report fasters grumbling of beginning results like crotchetiness, migraines, and distraction with hunger, they likewise say that after about a month, most fasters adjust and figure out how to endure the fasting way of life quite well. Thus, in light of this, beginning last November, I checked it out.

8-on 16-off

The primary technique I endeavored was the 8-on, 16-off strategy. As far as I might be concerned, this implied no food starting after supper (about 8pm) for 16 hours. I could eat again at about early afternoon the following day.

I attempted this strategy for seven days. I announced crotchetiness, migraines, and distraction with hunger. The most concerning issue with this strategy for me was that I'm a major breakfast eater. I like to awaken, work out, and eat. What's more, the initial two things on this rundown are much less propelling when the third isn't there. In spite of the fact that I got more used to the daily schedule before the week's over (I tackled the migraine issue by compelling myself to drink more water), the possibility of abandoning breakfast each day made me discouraged. What's more, despondency isn't useful for cerebrum wellbeing.

24 hours

So I chose to attempt the week by week 24-hour quick all things being equal. Along these lines, I contemplated, I could get the fasting over with in one shot. I began in late November, and have been fasting once every week, supper to-supper, since. I even figured out how to keep it up preposterous.

Results

Have I adjusted to my new way of life? All things considered, yes and no. I don't get cerebral pains, I'm normally not very surly on quick days, and in the event that I keep myself occupied I in every case quick on work days I can as a rule traverse the day without considering food. Be that as it may, abandoning nourishment for 24 hours is simply hard, and it seems like it will keep on being hard regardless of how often I do it. I did it yesterday, for the sixth or seventh time. It was hard.

In spite of the trouble, however, over the long run I've encountered an unforeseen response to my fasting schedule. I've come, unreasonably, to appreciate it. Furthermore, however mentally, I don't really anticipate my quick days, actually, I do. It's an inclination that is difficult to clarify, however in case you're a standard exerciser you may comprehend a relationship: it's like the craving you feel to get

84

up and get going subsequent to being stationary for an extensive stretch. Furthermore, when I'm through with a quick, to proceed with the activity relationship, I have a feeling that I do subsequent to completing an intense exercise: spent, yet cheerful. It's this startling response, which, it ends up, isn't strange, that has persuaded me that fasting is beneficial for me.

So in case you're pondering New Year's goals for physical and psychological wellness, I would suggest, in light of the science and my own insight, checking IER out. It can't do any harm on the off chance that you're keen about it, and it probably will assist you with building up a more grounded, better, body and cerebrum. Be that as it may, don't consider me answerable if, in the present moment at any rate, crotchetiness, cerebral pains, or distraction with food follow.

1.4 Irresistible Benefits of Intermittent Fasting for Your Brain
Intermittent fasting has gotten quite possibly the most well-known methodologies for getting in shape, and it's promoted as having numerous actual medical advantages. However, how can it deal with your cerebrum? We should bring a profound plunge into the exploration to discover what "time-confined eating" truly never really cerebrum.

Your Brain on
Intermittent Fasting

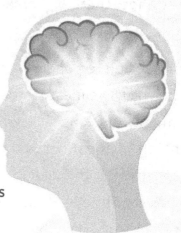

- Improved reasoning

- Increase in substances
  that promote growth
  of brain cells

- Improved communication
  between neurons

- Creation of new powerhouses
  in our brain cells

- Resistance to injury
  and disease

1. Triggers autophagy

Intermittent fasting turns on a significant interaction called autophagy, in which your mind "makes a garbage run" that develops during the day. This self-cleaning measure detoxifies the mind, get out old and harmed cells, and clear away garbage. This daily housekeeping advances the recovery of more up to date, better cells. An abundance of examination has shown that issues with autophagy have been connected to Alzheimer's sickness, despondency, bipolar turmoil, schizophrenia, and other neuropsychiatric problems.

2. Improves memory

Confining the hours when you eat has been appeared to essentially improve memory, as indicated by an investigation in the Journal of the Academy of Nutrition and Dietetics. In this examination, following a month of intermittent fasting, execution on a spatial arranging and working memory task and on a functioning memory limit test expanded altogether. Extra exploration on creatures has tracked down that intermittent fasting improves learning and memory.

3. Brightens mood

Exploration tracked down that following 3 months of intermittent fasting, study members announced improved states of mind and diminished strain, outrage, and disarray. Another examination from 2018 that was researching weight reduction methodologies tracked down that intermittent fasting was related with huge upgrades in enthusiastic prosperity and wretchedness.

4. Reduces inflammation

Constant aggravation has been connected to many cerebrum problems, including wretchedness, bipolar turmoil, over the top habitual issue (OCD), schizophrenia, Alzheimer's infection, and the sky is the limit from there. As per an investigation in Nutrition Research, intermittent fasting diminishes irritation, which can have powerful advantages for your mind wellbeing and mental prosperity.

5. Fights high blood sugar

Exploration shows that intermittent fasting produces more prominent enhancements in insulin affectability, which assists you with forestalling high glucose levels and type 2 diabetes. The diary Neurology has distributed discoveries showing that high glucose is related with a more modest hippocampus, the seahorse-molded design in your transient projections related with disposition, learning, and memory. Different investigations show that tension and sorrow are 2-3 times higher in patients with type 2 diabetes than everybody.

6. Lowers blood pressure at night

Intermittent fasting diminishes circulatory strain while you rest, which is advantageous for heart wellbeing, and anything that is useful for your heart is additionally useful for your cerebrum. Having hypertension or pre-hypertension brings blood stream down to the mind. Low blood stream on cerebrum SPECT imaging filters has been seen with gloom, bipolar confusion, schizophrenia, ADD/ADHD, horrendous mind injury, substance misuse, self-destructive contemplations, and then some. Also, low blood stream is the #1 mind imaging indicator that an individual will build up Alzheimer's infection.

7. Burns excess fat

Intermittent fasting assists with consuming more fat, which is useful for cerebrum wellbeing. Abundance fat on your body isn't your companion. A developing assortment of exploration, remembering reads for Archives of General Psychiatry and Psychosomatic Medicine, has discovered that heftiness is unfavorable to cerebrum wellbeing and is related with a more serious danger of melancholy, bipolar confusion, alarm issue, agoraphobia (dread of going out), and addictions.

With such a lot of examination highlighting significant mind medical advantages, you might need to join intermittent fasting into your way of life. What's the most ideal approach to do it? Quite possibly the most well-known techniques is to do a daily quick for 12-16 hours. The most straightforward approach to do it is to start fasting a few hours before sleep time. For instance, in the event that you have supper at 6 p.m., don't eat again until 6–10 a.m. the following day.

We adopt an entire body strategy to assisting individuals with defeating incapacitating manifestations and accomplish top execution. We perform extensive assessments that incorporate mind SPECT imaging, just as taking a gander at the numerous way of life factors, like eating regimen, that can add to emotional well-being indications or keep you away from arriving at your latent capacity. Our fold over administrations center on the most un-harmful, best arrangements, including mind wellbeing sustenance instructing.

1.5 Intermittent Fasting: How Does It Affect the Body and Brain?

Intermittent fasting is a mainstream sustenance pattern now, and I'm getting posed a great deal of inquiries about it. So I need to unload the science and give you my interpretation of it. Furthermore, on the off chance that you're pondering: indeed, I've attempted it actually and very like it however no, it isn't essential for our standard drug (more on why not underneath).

Essentially, individuals are utilizing Intermittent Fasting (or IF, for short) to get thinner, help diminish hypertension, help their asthma, and even oversee rheumatoid joint pain. It might likewise help secure against diabetes, coronary illness, and malignancy. Furthermore, it might even assistance you live more.

Also, obviously, there is a neuroscience point, as well. Intermittent fasting, or IF, may help your cerebrum in a couple of various ways. Who might have thought "un-powering" your cerebrum (just briefly, however!) can help it stay sound for more? We should have a glance at what the science is saying about the cerebrum boosting forces of intermittent fasting just as find solutions to a portion of my most every now and again posed inquiries on this subject.

Intermittent Fasting IF isn't an eating routine, yet rather an eating design that includes brief times of fasting. It doesn't prescribe what to eat, yet more so when to eat. Numerous individuals really discover intermittent fasting IF simple to follow on the grounds that eating less dinners in a more limited time span can improve on their life. Notwithstanding, in the event that you have glucose issues (and the greater part of our customers in the cerebrum and psychological wellness space do!) at that point intermittent fasting IF isn't for you, until we get you off the glucose rollercoaster. Got that? We don't need any hypoglycemia (for example low glucose) or ensuing swooning, in the event that you attempt IF when you have glucose issues.

Due to the confined eating times, intermittent fasting IF lessens the measure of calories burned-through for brief timeframes. Consequently the "un-powering" angle. This aides drive the body and cerebrum medical advantages. Another impact is that IF helps consume fat. At the point when your body doesn't get enough calories from food, it utilizes the calories put away as fat.

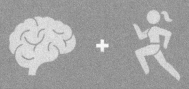

FOR YOUR BRAIN AND BODY

Intermittent fasting expands your digestion, decreases your danger of coronary illness, and lessens both oxidation and irritation. Fasting likewise influences your chemicals in a manner that lessens glucose and improves insulin obstruction. In the event that builds your digestion, decreases your danger of coronary illness, and lessens both oxidation and aggravation. Also that (in creature examines, up until this point) it can likewise lessen the danger of diabetes, malignancy, and even broaden life expectancy.

Intermittent fasting likewise helps in diminishing oxidation (for example free extremists), decreasing aggravation (counting that awful neuro-inflammation), and balancing out glucose levels likewise advantage your mind.

How precisely does IF help your cerebrum? I thought you'd never inquire! Here are the main 5 different ways, as upheld by the neuroscience research.

1. Intermittent fasting: For more brain proteins

One of the primary ways IF benefits the mind is by expanding one of my number one proteins that the cerebrum makes, mind determined neurotropic factor (BDNF). I love BDNF on the grounds that it is useful to synapses by being a development factor. It develops new neurons (nerve/synapses), permits them to converse with each other, and is a characteristic stimulant. In creature considers, BDNF additionally assists neurons with remaining better more and assists them with opposing basic cerebrum sicknesses (like dementia) and injury (from strokes). All by keeping up legitimate neuron construction and capacity.

2. Intermittent fasting may aid in the development of new nerve cells.

Intermittent fasting really assists with developing new nerve cells. Serious fasting brings about a decrease in size in many organs with the exception of the cerebrum. You definitely realized your body puts forth an admirable attempt to safeguard your super significant noggin, correct? (If it's not too much trouble, note that I'm not discussing "serious fasting" with IF.)

Indeed, mammalian cerebrums develop new nerve cells when intermittently fasting! All in all, how accomplishes more cerebrum chemical and new nerve cells convert into better neuron-wellbeing, you inquire? All things considered, they assist with cerebrum maturing, mind harm from strokes, and epilepsy. Here's the means by which (and I'm so energized for this part!).

3. Intermittent fasting for healthier ageing of the brain

Intermittent fasting appears to keep our minds remaining more youthful. It might even ensure against neurodegeneration (loss of design and capacity of neurons) from Alzheimer's illness, Parkinson's infection and Huntington's sickness. One little investigation, for instance, showed that IF improved intellectual (capacity to think) in individuals with psychological debilitation. Ten individuals with early indications of Alzheimer's begun a few way of life upgrades including a 12-hour quick every evening. Inside 3-6 months, nine of the ten patients had improved comprehension. Preclinical creature concentrates likewise show that IF may postpone the beginning, or lessen seriousness of Alzheimer's, Parkinson's, and Huntington's sicknesses.

4. Intermittent fasting can help prevent stroke-related brain injury.

Studies show that creatures who get strokes have less cerebrum harm on the off chance that they've been intermittently fasting. They likewise have more BDNF alongside cell reinforcement and calming mind compounds.

Likewise, in addition to the fact that they had less mind harm, however less of them passed on in light of the stroke. I think this is significant examination since it recommends that IF might actually secure us against both mind harm and passing from suffering a heart attack.

5. Epilepsy and intermittent fasting

Numerous investigations show that when a mind utilizes less of its fundamental fuel, sugars, as it does in the fasting state (and the ketogenic diet), the quantity of epileptic seizures decreases. Strangely, while both the ketogenic diet and IF appear to lessen seizures, the sorts of seizures that each decreased were unique. More examination is required around here.

1.7 Best 2 Methods of Intermittent Fasting for Healthier Brain

There are a couple of basic approaches to intermittently quick and I have by and by tried two of the most ideal ways on myself. I very like IF (yet once more, I can't say sufficiently this: on the off chance that you're riding that glucose thrill ride please get off it before you endeavor intermittent fasting).

Method 1:

A few group eat every one of their calories inside 8 hours of the day, fasting for the other 16 hours. This can work, for instance, by skipping breakfast and eating just between 12:00 p.m. until 8:00 p.m. During the fasting period, you can drink water, coffee (only one, please, and of good quality), or tea, as long as they are sugar-free.

Method 2:

Another approach to do IF is by eating regularly five days of the week. On two non-back to back days that week, eat close to 600 calories. For individuals who start IF, there is a progress time of 3 a month and a half. During this time the body and cerebrum adjust to the new eating example, and I discover a few group even notification improved temperament.

One late examination says, "We infer that there is extraordinary potential for ways of life that join occasional fasting during grown-up life to advance ideal wellbeing and decrease the danger of numerous constant sicknesses, especially for the individuals who are overweight and stationary." In my assessment however, IF isn't for everybody (I think this will be my third time saying it so hear me! Fix your hypoglycemia before you attempt intermittent fasting!)

On the off chance that ought to likewise be stayed away from in youngsters, the old, and grown-ups who are underweight. We likewise realize that it tends to be unsafe for individuals with certain ailments, for example, amyotrophic horizontal sclerosis. Indeed, even as a sound grown-up there might be times when IF makes you very ravenous, or truly and intellectually exhausted. Assuming you endeavor IF a couple of times and over and over feel truly messy, simply eat (a complex carb with a fat or protein). On the off chance that could very well not be ideal for you right now, and you can attempt it again in a couple of months.

My input on IF is that it's a helpful method of eating with some great arising proof to back it up. Like I said, I've attempted it and like it (however I've likewise gone through years chipping away at fixing my glucose). Be that as it may, I'm reluctant to prescribe it to customers as a feature of their prescription on the grounds that, while the science is cool, that far is generally in rodents or minuscule examples with people. Be that as it may, I think if your glucose is steady, and you're truly tingling to attempt it, at that point give it a go. Attempt one of the manners in which I suggest above and check whether it's something that works for you.

Chapter 2. Intermittent Fasting as a Therapy in Neurological Disease

Intermittent fasting is profoundly settled in development, yet its possible applications to the present generally normal, handicapping neurological illnesses remain moderately neglected. Intermittent Fasting incites a changed metabolic express that upgrades neuron bioenergetics, versatility, and strength in a way that may check an expansive cluster of neurological problems. In the two creatures and people, intermittent fasting forestalls and treats the metabolic condition, a significant danger factor for some neurological sicknesses. In creatures, intermittent fasting most likely forestalls the development of tumors, conceivably treats set up tumors, and improves tumor reactions to chemotherapy. In human malignancies, including tumors that include the cerebrum, intermittent fasting improves chemotherapy-related unfavorable impacts and may shield ordinary cells from chemotherapy. Intermittent fasting improves insight, slows down age-related psychological decrease, for the most part eases back neurodegeneration, diminishes cerebrum harm and upgrades practical recuperation after stroke, and mitigates the neurotic and clinical highlights of epilepsy and different sclerosis in creature models. Essentially because of an absence of exploration, the proof supporting intermittent fasting as a treatment in human neurological problems, including neurodegeneration, stroke, epilepsy, and numerous sclerosis, is backhanded or non-existent. Given the strength of the creature proof, many energizing revelations may lie ahead, anticipating future examinations concerning the feasibility of intermittent fasting as a treatment in neurological infection.

2.1 Introduction

Intermittent fasting has flooded in fame over the new thousand years. Quite a bit of its newly discovered eagerness has been driven by a developing public insight that intermittent fasting might be advantageous for some parts of human wellbeing. In spite of the implied medical advantages of intermittent fasting, it remains to some degree unfamiliar to ordinary clinical practice, albeit the present circumstance isn't by and large new; intermittent fasting has truly fallen all through style in its relationship to medication. As Mark Twain may have said, "History doesn't rehash the same thing, however it rhymes."

To get why and how intermittent fasting might be pertinent as a treatment to a variety of neurological illnesses, it is useful to analyze intermittent fasting in both transformative and unthinking settings. In doing as such, it should progressively become obvious that intermittent fasting and drug based methodologies need not be totally unrelated; they can be joined, and such a methodology may really be ideal. In a time of rising medical care costs and an expanding predominance of handicapping neurological issues, the effect of a self-engaging, sans cost, viable treatment close by ordinary clinical methodologies would be significant and positive.

On this foundation, the definition, roots, instruments, and different regimens of intermittent fasting are talked about, trailed by a rundown of the proof supporting intermittent fasting in the avoidance and treatment of an assortment of neurological issues, followed ultimately by a talk on the most widely recognized unfavorable impacts and confusions related with intermittent fasting.

2.2 Pre-Human Evolutionary Origins of Intermittent Fasting

"Intermittent Fasting" might be characterized as a deliberate restraint from food and drink for determined, repeating timeframes, with the intermittent fasting time frames ordinarily going from 12 hours to three weeks in people. Intermittent Fasting is frequently stood out from not obligatory ("as wanted") taking care of, which is portrayed by at least three dinners each day in present day cultures, and joined with a stationary way of life may expand an individual's danger of building up an ongoing neurological sickness. Intermittent Fasting ought not to be mistaken for starvation, a condition of ongoing dietary inadequacy which is neither intentional nor controlled, and which may come full circle in organ disappointment and passing.

In development, living beings ready to endure conditions without supplements for broadened timeframes held a significant endurance advantage over those unfit to do as such. The transformative determination strain to endure the burdens related with low-energy conditions has delivered various intermittent fasting-incited metabolic systems that have been moderated for millions, if not billions, of years in people

Many single-celled and straightforward multicellular life forms change their digestion during seasons of supplement shortage, the point of which is to preserve assets, limit harm, and upgrade life span. For instance, when freak Escherichia coli microbes are moved from a supplement rich stock to a sans calorie medium, they go through a progression of metabolic changes that permit them to endure multiple times longer than wild-type microorganisms, and when the yeast Saccharomyces is traded from a development medium to water, it enters a fixed stage that expands its pressure resilience and pairs its life expectancy. Comparable reactions have likewise been seen in basic multicellular life forms denied of supplements, like the nematode, which changes to a metabolic "dauer state," bringing about a generous expansion in life expectancy.

Past these more straightforward living things, various complex multicellular living beings, like lungfish, eels, frogs, snakes, and arthropods, have likewise advanced unprecedented protections from supplement shortage, halfway due to diminished resting metabolic rates and movement levels. Notwithstanding, as opposed to enter a lethargic stage, some unpredictable organic entities really increment their intellectual and actual work levels when abstained, improving their capacity to look for and obtain food. Rodents on a

104

intermittent fasting routine, for instance, have shown diminishes in the size of most organs, beside the cerebrum (and balls), bringing about kept up or improved psychological and actual execution. In another model, hostage lions changed from a traditional every day taking care of timetable to a "chasm and quick" plan comprising of just three dinners each week have shown a decrease in maladaptive, stereotypic practices, like pacing, and an increment in versatile, chasing related practices, for example, sniffing and following.

In the same way as other of the living beings that went before them in advancement, pre-agrarian people persevered through ordinary times of food shortage. People have been tracker finders for a very long time; it was just a moderately short 12,000 years prior that the progress to horticulture happened. Hence, post-horticultural people might not have had adequate opportunity to completely adjust to the ceaseless food supply given by cultivating, which may to some degree clarify the later presentation of willful intermittent fasting rehearses by most of civilizations on earth. The old Romans, for instance, accepted that eating more than one huge dinner each day was unfortunate. Most world religions, including Christianity and Islam, likewise joined normal fasting into their strict practices.

In more current occasions, the potential medical advantages of intermittent fasting have been intermittently perceived and neglected. The American doctor Edward Dewey embraced a to some degree extremist perspective on intermittent fasting during the 1800s, accepting that basically all infection originated from inordinate eating. During the 1900s, German doctor, the principal individual to thoroughly report the advantageous impacts of intermittent fasting in numerous human illnesses, composed that "intermittent fasting is, no doubt, the best organic strategy for treatment". An Italian-conceived bio gerontologist and intermittent fasting specialist during the 2000s, has as of late recommended that intermittent fasting specifically enacts numerous "life span programs" which may lead not exclusively to an all-inclusive life expectancy, yet additionally to an all-encompassing wellbeing length. Inquisitively, regardless of these and other intermittent fasting advocates, the set up eating design in most current cultures stays at least three suppers each day, an example that is related with an internationally expanding predominance of corpulence, type 2 diabetes, and an assortment of debilitating neurological issues.

2.3 Intermittent Fasting: Mechanisms

Intermittent fasting initiates the planned modification of numerous metabolic and transcriptional instruments that may impact neurons. Altogether, these modifications produce an entire body, changed metabolic express that upgrades neuron bioenergetics, pliancy, and strength to push, coming full circle in kept up or even improved intellectual execution.

Intermittent Fasting: A Whole-Body, Altered Metabolic State

Following 12–36 hours of intermittent fasting, the human body enters a physiological condition of ketosis described by low blood glucose levels, depleted liver glycogen stores, and the hepatic creation of fat-determined ketone bodies, or ketones, which fill in as a significant fuel hotspot for the cerebrum. The liver is the essential site of ketogenesis, however cerebrum astrocytes additionally produce ketones. Inside a few days of starting a quick, ketones become the cerebrum's favored fuel source, giving up to 70% of its energy necessities. Ketones comprise a more proficient wellspring of energy per unit oxygen in muscles, and perhaps in the cerebrum, upgrading neuron bioenergetics and psychological execution; for instance, it has been shown that rodents exposed to a ketone ester for five days display improved spatial learning and memory.

However ketones are something beyond a fuel hotspot for neurons; the essential blood ketone, (BHB), additionally serves significant flagging capacities. In hippocampal and cortical neurons, BHB plays an essential flagging job by instigating the record of mind determined neurotropic factor (BDNF) by means of its hindrance of histone deacetylases, compounds that subdue BDNF articulation. BDNF is a vital controller of neuron work; it animates mitochondria biogenesis, keeps up synaptic design, spikes the creation and endurance of new hippocampal neurons, and upgrades neuron protection from injury and illness.

Notwithstanding BHB and BDNF, intermittent fasting incites the statement of an expert controller of mitochondria, the record factor peroxisome proliferator-initiated receptor. It is a focal inducer of mitochondria biogenesis, expanding mitochondria biomass, which thusly upgrades neuron bioenergetics and empowers synaptic pliancy. It likewise balances the creation and capacity of mitochondria; for instance, muscle mitochondria segregated from transgenic mice that ectopically express it show an expanded respiratory limit contrasted with wild-type controls. Accordingly, it isn't just invigorates mitochondria biogenesis, it additionally animates the development of mitochondria with modified natural properties; both have a constructive outcome on neuron bioenergetics.

Intermittent fasting shows powerful impacts on glucose digestion and insulin flagging. In people, intermittent fasting for three-to-five days diminishes blood glucose levels by 30%–40%, and hinders glycolysis. Intermittent fasting on substitute days for three weeks diminishes insulin levels by half 60% on the abstained day. When all is said in done, three-to-five days of intermittent fasting in people additionally brings about a 60% decrease in insulin-like development factor, the central development factor in warm blooded animals, a five-to-ten times expansion in restricting protein,

108

one of its principle restricting proteins, and a few overlay expansion in development chemical (GH), which ascends to protect bulk. Intermittent fasting along these lines forestalls the improvement of persistent, extreme, and possibly dysregulated glucose digestion while simultaneously saving insulin affectability and development factor flagging, all of which may profit neuron bioenergetics.

Intermittent fasting additionally applies an amazing impact cell union and corruption measures. The equilibrium of cell amalgamation versus corruption is controlled by the particular exercises of two expert controllers of digestion, mammalian objective of rapamycin and AMP-initiated protein kinase. Under high-supplement conditions (especially amino acids), it animates protein union and cell development; conversely, when cell energy holds are low, AMPK down manages it to limit energy utilization and invigorate autophagy, an intracellular corruption pathway that clears not collapsed proteins and harmed organelles, reuses supplements, and reinforces energy creation. Intermittent fasting smothers it and raises AMPK, in this manner restricting supplement utilization and development for autophagy and endurance; despite the fact that AMPK have generally been concentrated in muscle cells, ongoing proof proposes these two adversarial ace metabolic controllers may likewise intercede intermittent fasting reactions in neurons.

Intermittent Fasting impacts fat digestion by adjusting the hormonal exercises of leptin, adiponectin, and ghrelin. Leptin is related with a favorable to fiery state, though adiponectin is related with upgraded insulin affectability and stifled irritation. Ghrelin is likewise connected with upgraded insulin affectability; additionally, ghrelin may animate hippocampal synaptic versatility and neurogenesis. Intermittent fasting diminishes leptin however builds adiponectin and ghrelin, changes that are likely helpful for neuron bioenergetics and the support of neural pathways.

Finally, intermittent fasting stifles irritation, lessening the outflow of favorable to fiery cytokines like interleukin 6 (IL6) and tumor rot factor. Since provocative cycles support a wide range of neurological problems, the capacity of intermittent fasting to smother neural and fundamental aggravation may improve neuron endurance in these issues.

Intermittent Fasting: More than just Calorie Restriction in Brain Development

Calorie limitation alludes to a constant 20%–40% decrease in calorie consumption, with feast recurrence kept up. Longer than a hundred years of examination has shown that calorie limitation diminishes persistent illness and protracts life expectancy in an assortment of animal groups. Since calorie limitation and intermittent fasting share numerous comparative instruments and intermittent fasting regularly creates a reduction in calorie admission after some time, the inquiry is frequently raised concerning whether the possible advantages of intermittent fasting are only because of decreased calorie consumption, rather than a specific impact of the intermittent fasting.

A few examinations in creatures and people have demonstrated that intermittent fasting may present advantages on cell (counting neuron) digestion past calorie limitation. It has been shown that a few mice abstained on substitute days can eat twice as much on the taking care of day, to such an extent that their net week after week calorie admission stays like mice took care of not indispensable; notwithstanding the absence of by and large calorie limitation, the previous still presentation helpful metabolic impacts contrasted with the last mentioned, including improved glucose levels and insulin movement, just as upgraded neuron protection from a neurotoxin, kainic corrosive. Studies including overweight and hefty non-diabetic people have shown more noteworthy enhancements in insulin affectability in abstained people contrasted with their non-abstained, calorie-coordinated with partners. As of late, a five-week randomized hybrid preliminary in men with pre-diabetes analyzed a intermittent fasting routine, containing adequate by and large calorie admission to forestall weight reduction, against a benchmark group with a customary eating plan; albeit the two gatherings were coordinated for calorie consumption, the intermittent fasting bunch showed more noteworthy upgrades in insulin affectability and different proportions of metabolic wellbeing.

HOW INTERMITTENT FASTING EFFECTS THE BRAIN

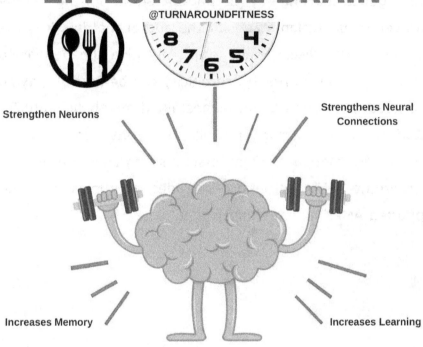

@TURNAROUNDFITNESS

Strengthen Neurons

Strengthens Neural Connections

Increases Memory

Increases Learning

The clearest clarification for a putative, fasting-explicit impact on metabolic wellbeing may lie in the principal qualification between intermittent fasting and calorie limitation timing. In particular, fasting is applied intermittently, while calorie limitation is nonstop. Following 12–36 hours of intermittent fasting, there is a perceivable metabolic change or "switch" from using sugars and glucose to unsaturated fats and ketones as the major cell fuel sources. During the abstained express, the switch is "on," hypothetically up managing autophagy and endurance pathways in neurons, while during the fed express, the switch is "off," stressing redesigning and development pathways. Hence, in contrast to calorie limitation, intermittent fasting benefits from each consecutive bioenergetics challenge by "setting the stage" for a generally calm cell recuperation stage; at the end of the day, it is the exchanging the discontinuity that may give the benefit to neuron digestion. In reality, chronicity can be hurtful, paying little heed to a took care of or abstained metabolic state for instance, intense trigger initiation advances muscle hypertrophy, though constant enactment produces decay, and intermittent AMPK actuation upgrades neuroplasticity, yet supported AMPK initiation disables it.

Three boundaries describe an intermittent fasting routine the power of the food and drink limitation, the recurrence of the intermittent fasting time frames, and the term of the intermittent fasting time frames. The "ideal" intermittent fasting routine relies upon singular way of life and decency.

Intensity of the Food and Drink Restriction in IF

The "power" of a quick alludes to the sum and sort of food and drink that might be allowed during the intermittent fasting time frames. The force of an intermittent fasting period goes from the total oversight of all food and drink (an "unadulterated" quick) to a negligible admission of explicit suppers pointed toward keeping up the abstained metabolic state.

Diets that wipe out all food and drink are adroitly straightforward, however from a functional point of view, the absence of water consumption forces a practical most extreme maximum constraint of 24 hours. An illustration of this sort of quick happens during the Islamic month of Ramadan, where people avoid all food and drink from dawn to nightfall, for roughly 30 days.

Water-just diets exclude all calorie allow yet give satisfactory hydration and can subsequently be stretched out to a few days, weeks, or even months, given that sufficient salt and different micronutrients are kept up. Liquid just diets furthermore grant without calorie liquids, like tea and dark espresso, which can help keep up energy and smother the transient rushes of yearning that may happen in certain individuals. The two kinds of diets should focus on at least 2–2.5 L of water or liquid admission each day, and a multivitamin might be added to give micronutrients.

For people who experience issues enduring liquid just diets, a level of intermittent fasting power can be traded for improved bearableness utilizing explicit feast decisions that don't upset the abstained metabolic state. The caloric admission of these suppers ought not to surpass 250–500 kcal each day. One normal alternative is to consolidate an everyday vegetable or bone stock into the quick, which additionally gives liquids and micronutrients.

Frequency and Duration of the Intermittent Fasting Periods

Most strains of mice can't get by for over three days without food, yet most people can endure intermittent fasting times of 30 days or more. Given this capacity too quick for expanded time spans, considerable fluctuation exists in the recurrence and term of fasting regimens accessible to people.

The most okay of all intermittent fasting regimens might be time-limited taking care of (TRF), which comprises of every day intermittent fasting periods enduring 12–20 hours, rotating with a day by day four-to-twelve hour "eating window". There is some proof that limiting the eating window to the morning or center of the day produces prevalent impacts on muscle to fat ratio and insulin opposition contrasted with late evening or evening eating windows.

Intermittent Fasting periods enduring longer than a day are frequently gathered under the comprehensively utilized term "intermittent fasting," the meaning of which regularly fluctuates relying upon the source. From a viable perspective, it is most likely best to utilize hold the utilization of this term for intermittent fasting regimens containing repeating intermittent fasting periods enduring 24–48 hours in length. In human examinations, the most well-known intermittent fasting regimens are substitute every day fasting (ADF) and intermittent fasting for two successive days out of each week (two-days-of the week intermittent fasting).

Occasional intermittent fasting regularly alludes to expanded intermittent fasting periods enduring from two days to three weeks in length. Occasional fasting may deliver more articulated metabolic changes contrasted with TRF, ADF, or two-days-out of every week intermittent fasting; in any case, for some individuals, intermittent fasting is hard to endure and may not be fundamental, contingent upon a person's objectives. Intermittent Fasting periods enduring a while to longer than a year have been recorded in people, yet these address excellent cases.

Evidence Supporting Intermittent Fasting in Neurological Disease

Intermittent Fasting may defer maturing, a significant danger factor for neurological sickness. Past maturing, convincing proof in creatures and people has shown that intermittent fasting can forestall and treat the metabolic condition, another significant danger factor for an assortment of neurological infections. Intermittent fasting can likewise forestall and treat numerous neurological problems in creatures; because of an absence of exploration, significantly less proof is accessible in people. More human investigations are required.

2.5 Metabolic Syndrome during Intermittent Fasting

The metabolic condition comprises of a blend of stomach corpulence, insulin obstruction, hypertension, and dyslipidemia. Intermittent fasting lightens the critical intermittent ties of the metabolic condition in creatures and people, bringing about valuable impacts that are comparable and at times better than those saw with calorie limitation.

Intermittent Fasting as a Therapy in the Metabolic Syndrome

Intermittent fasting reliably mitigates stoutness in creature models. Rodents kept up on intermittent fasting regimens show lower body loads contrasted with rodents took care of not indispensable, with long haul (more than 20 weeks) intermittent fasting regimens for the most part delivering huge weight reduction. In addition, the lower body loads to a great extent result from decreased fat mass, not fit mass; the last is saved.

In creatures, intermittent fasting regimens additionally destroy instinctive fat and improve insulin affectability. Intermittent fasting fixes type 2 diabetes in rat models, an impact that isn't because of calorie limitation given that TRF creatures burn-through similar by and large calories as creatures took care of not obligatory, yet the previous presentation an enemy of diabetic impact though the last don't. In certain examinations, intermittent fasting regimens have prompted advantageous consequences for insulin obstruction that are better than those incited by even serious calorie limitation; for instance, rodents on ADF can keep up comparative body loads contrasted with rodents took care of not obligatory, yet the previous still show enhancements in glucose levels and insulin movement that are just about as

119

extraordinary as, or more prominent than, those exhibited by rodents on a 40% calorie limitation.

ADF diminishes pulse and circulatory strain in rodents in no time, with both proceeding to diminish until settling at lower levels before a month's over, after which they stay low on both intermittent fasting and taking care of days. Rodents on an ADF routine likewise show expansions in pulse changeability, just as better cardiovascular variation than an immobilization stress. The fasting-intervened consequences for pulse, circulatory strain, pulse changeability, and cardiovascular pressure transformation are thought to result from expansions in BDNF, which improves the cholinergic action of brainstem cardio vagal neurons. They don't have all the earmarks of being intervened by calorie limitation, given that rodents on ADF, with a generally speaking 10%–20% calorie limitation, show more prominent declines in resting pulse than rodents kept up on a persistent 40% calorie limitation.

The proof for intermittent fasting-incited weight reduction in people isn't just about as reliable as in creatures; be that as it may, present moment (under a half year) intermittent fasting regimens by and large lead to weight reduction in overweight and hefty people. Numerous individuals going through strict diets experience weight reduction, however it is frequently recaptured a while later. Alternately, audits of overweight and fat individuals set on two-to half year intermittent fasting regimens by and large exhibit a 3%–16% decrease in body weight contrasted with controls, with regimens more than a quarter of a year bound to show a clinically significant weight decrease of 5 kg or more. Both intermittent fasting and calorie limitation regimens produce comparative levels of weight reduction, albeit a few examinations recommend that intermittent fasting regimens might be better than a 20%–25% calorie limitation. In addition, notwithstanding comparable abatements in body weight, intermittent fasting might be more powerful than calorie limitation at holding slender mass.

Intermittent fasting has been known to turn around type 2 diabetes in people for above and beyond a century, frequently wiping out the requirement for diabetic meds. Additionally, intermittent fasting regimens seem to apply insulin-sharpening impacts autonomous of weight reduction, and non-diabetic and pre-diabetic people going through intermittent fasting regimens show more noteworthy upgrades in insulin affectability contrasted with non-abstained people coordinated for calorie admission. On the whole, these discoveries propose that the insulin-sharpening impacts of intermittent fasting are, in any event somewhat, autonomous of weight reduction and calorie limitation.

In people, six-to-24 weeks of ADF or two-days-out of every week intermittent fasting incites a critical diminishing in pulse (3%–8% systolic and 6%–10% diastolic), for the most part with regards to weight reduction. Occasional fasting is especially viable at diminishing circulatory strain in hypertensive people; systolic pulse falls by 20–60 mmHg inside one-to about fourteen days. Intermittent Fasting and calorie limitation show comparable consequences for circulatory strain decrease.

2.6 Neurodegeneration

Neurodegenerative problems, like Huntington's infection (HD), Parkinson's illness (PD), and Alzheimer's sickness (AD), distress various neurons (striatal barbed neurons in HD, boundless dopaminergic and cholinergic neurons in PD, and cortical cholinergic neurons in AD); nonetheless, every one of the three issues show impeded neuron bioenergetics, glucose digestion, and neurotropic factor flagging. In each of the three, there is a decreased articulation of the expert mitochondria controller, alongside a related decrease in mitochondria biogenesis and capacity. In addition, the respiratory chain is weakened in PD and AD, particularly PD, which exhibits a checked shortage at complex I. Moreover, both PD and AD show disabilities in neuron glucose digestion and insulin flagging, particularly AD, which is portrayed by cerebrum insulin insufficiency just as opposition, consequently prompting AD being depicted as a type of mind explicit, "type 3" diabetes.

Intermittent Fasting as a Therapy in Neurodegeneration

Intermittent Fasting improves perception and forestalls psychological decrease in non-neurodegenerative creature models. Rodents on intermittent fasting regimens show upgraded psychological execution contrasted with those took care of not obligatory. TRF slows down age-related decreases in cerebrum white matter honesty, energy creation, and comprehension saw in rodents took care of not obligatory. Mice kept up on TRF additionally show expanded hippocampal BDNF levels, synaptic strength, and neurogenesis, proposing that the upgrades in comprehension are, somewhat, intervened by BDNF.

Intermittent fasting typically eases back neurodegeneration in creature models of HD, PD, and AD. Huntington freak mice show lacks in striatal and cortical BDNF levels just as glucose digestion, trailed by neurodegeneration and engine brokenness; nonetheless, if ADF is started early enough, BDNF levels increment, glucose digestion standardizes, and neurodegeneration and engine brokenness are postponed. In PD mouse models, ADF gives insurance against the dopaminergic neuron degeneration and misfortune instigated by the mitochondria poison (MPTP), bringing about improved useful results contrasted with mice took care of ad libitum feed. Since MPTP meddles with complex I of the mitochondria respiratory chain, this helpful impact may part of the way be because of the ketones created by intermittent fasting, which hypothetically bypass the PD complex I imperfection through an unpredictable II-subordinate instrument, upgrading mitochondria bioenergetics. In AD mouse models, ADF has been appeared to present expanded hippocampal neuron protection from the neurotoxic impacts of kainic corrosive, bringing about improved intellectual execution, and ADF enhances age-related psychological shortfalls that happen in transgenic mice communicating beta-amyloid forerunner protein, presenilin 1, and tau changes.

Until this point, intermittent fasting has not been investigated as a treatment in individuals with HD, PD, and AD. In any case, roundabout proof has been given by investigations of ketogenic abstains from food in these problems. Ketogenic abstains from food are high-fat, satisfactory protein, low-sugar slims down that power the body to consume fats as opposed to carbs as the essential fuel source, hence imitating an abstained metabolic state by creating ketones and initiating a significant number of the metabolic instruments actuated by intermittent fasting. In Parkinson's disease, a small case study found improved engine symptoms after a month on a ketogenic diet, and a subsequent randomized controlled trial involving 47 people with mild to severe PD found improvements in a significant number of the most disabling, least levodopa-responsive PD nonmotor side effects after two months on a ketogenic diet. Concerns about the ketogenic diet's effects. Concerning impacts of a ketogenic diet in AD, a solitary case arrangement including 15 individuals with gentle to-direct AD detailed gentle enhancements in discernment following 12 weeks of such an eating routine; these discoveries might be incompletely clarified by the way that despite the fact that mind glucose take-up is notably hindered in AD, ketone usage isn't.

2.7 Stroke

A stroke is a neurological shortfall of abrupt beginning because of an interfered with blood supply, bringing about mind, spinal string, or retinal dead tissue. Most strokes overall are ischemic and include neuron misfortune, neuroinflammation, neural organization reworking, and neuron utilitarian revamping.

Intermittent Fasting as a Therapy in Stroke

In creatures, intermittent fasting preceding an ischemic stroke reduces mind harm and improves practical recuperation. Rodents kept up on ADF preceding impediment of the center cerebral conduit show less mind harm and improved practical results contrasted with those took care of not indispensable. Additionally, mice kept up on TRF for a quarter of a year preceding center cerebral course impediment show expanded neurogenesis in the hippocampus and sub ventricular zones, just as infarcts not exactly a large portion of the size of those found in mice took care of not obligatory. Besides, rodents kept up on TRF for a quarter of a year prior and 70 days after worldwide cerebral ischemia show steady upgrades in spatial memory contrasted with non-intermittent fasting controls. The impacts of intermittent fasting after an ischemic stroke has effectively happened are not known, albeit roundabout proof is accessible from horrible mind and spinal rope examines which show that the execution of a intermittent fasting routine after a horrendous cerebrum injury presents neuroprotection and improves useful recuperation. Beforehand, it has been shown that harmed rodent cortex displays a striking, 8.5-overlay expansion in BHB take-up contrasted with trick creatures, which recommends that a significant part of the intermittent fasting-intervened recuperation in ischemic stroke might be because of the expanded metabolic effectiveness of BHB contrasted with glucose. Nonetheless, all things considered, up directed BDNF, upgraded mitochondria work, initiated pressure reaction flagging pathways, and smothered neuroinflammation likewise assume significant parts.

Human examinations on the immediate impacts of intermittent fasting in ischemic stroke are inadequate. Be that as it may, intermittent fasting lessens levels of supportive of fiery elements, for example, C-receptive protein, IL6, and homocysteine, which may hinder the arrangement of atherosclerotic plaques, a typical wellspring of stroke in people.

2.8 Epilepsy

Epilepsy is described by neuron hyper volatility, prompting a suffering inclination to produce seizures. In spite of a variety of hostile to epileptic medications and the accessibility of medical procedure, 33% of individuals with epilepsy keep on encountering drug-safe seizures.

Intermittent Fasting as a Therapy in Epilepsy

Unassuming proof backings intermittent fasting for seizure control in creature models of epilepsy. Contrasted with mice took care of not obligatory, mice on TRF show a delayed inertness to seizure age and a decline in the seriousness and recurrence of seizures. A particularly against seizure impact is in any event halfway because of the immediate anticonvulsant impacts of BHB. In any case, intermittent fasting may furthermore give seizure insurance by modifying the exercises of metabolic factors like IGF, and AMPK.

Intermittent fasting has been utilized to treat epilepsy since the time of Hippocrates, yet it was not until 1911 that it was officially archived the adequacy of intermittent fasting in the treatment of 20 individuals with epilepsy. With the presentation of Wilder's ketogenic diet and a long progression of hostile to epileptic medications, practically no investigations of intermittent fasting in epilepsy were distributed for almost a century. As of late, a little report explored the impacts of a two-month altered TRF routine in six epileptic kids with a deficient reaction to a ketogenic diet, announcing that four of the six kids experienced unassuming enhancements in seizure control. These outcomes are to be expected, as intermittent fasting and ketogenic counts calories share numerous comparative components; for instance, both increment BHB, which in certain examinations has related with improved seizure control, and both prompt extra instruments that altogether settle synaptic capacity. In any case, since a portion of the abstained kids experienced humble upgrades in seizure control past those of a ketogenic diet, there might be significant contrasts in the counter seizure instruments hidden intermittent fasting and ketogenic slims down.

2.9 Multiple Sclerosis

Different sclerosis (MS) is a provocative, immune system intervened jumble that harms focal sensory system neurons and their axons. As of late, there has been an expanding center around the part of gut microorganisms and their metabolites in MS, given that both are significant controllers of T cell separation and enteric safe reactions. This proposes that dietary components, which apply a solid impact on gut miniature biota creation and metabolite creation, may add to the pathogenesis of MS.

Intermittent Fasting as a Therapy in Multiple Sclerosis

Intermittent Fasting is valuable in exploratory immune system encephalomyelitis (EAE), a creature model of MS that includes the fiery intervened demyelination and passing of oligodendrocytes. In mice, ADF improves the neurotic and clinical highlights of EAE, upgrades gut microorganisms' variety, and increments administrative T cell numbers. Besides, fecal miniature biota moves from ADF mice to mice took care of not obligatory lessening the seriousness of EAE in the last mentioned, showing that a portion of the advantages of intermittent fasting might be interceded by gut microorganisms. Substituting patterns of a intermittent fasting-imitating diet (FMD), which copies intermittent fasting by giving a standard measure of food seriously diminished in calorie thickness, additionally lessen the clinical seriousness of EAE in mice, remembering a total inversion of manifestations for 20% of them. Potential systems hidden the FMD in EAE incorporate upgraded oligodendrocyte antecedent cell recovery and axon remyelination, just as improved guideline of immune system cells and favorable to incendiary markers.

Intermittent fasting holds guarantee as a treatment in human provocative intervened infections, despite the fact that there is no immediate proof supporting it as a treatment in MS. Intermittent Fasting produces obsessive and clinical enhancements in non-neurological, incendiary intervened sicknesses, like rheumatoid joint pain and asthma. As to, a pilot preliminary including 17 individuals with backsliding dispatching MS tracked down that an adjusted intermittent fasting routine actuated changes suggestive of those found in rat EAE models, including comparative, potentially helpful modifications to the gut miniature biota. The FMD may likewise improve the clinical and personal satisfaction scores in individuals with backsliding transmitting MS.

2.10 Challenges to Implementing Intermittent Fasting in Neurological Disease

To appropriately apply intermittent fasting as a treatment in neurological sickness, it is fundamental to perceive when intermittent fasting could conceivably be shown, realize how to oversee regular unfavorable impacts that may happen, and know about a few basic confusions.

Potential Contraindications

Not all people are appropriate for intermittent fasting, and surprisingly the most reasonable up-and-comers may create intermittent fasting-related unfriendly impacts. Most antagonistic impacts can be tried not to by guarantee sufficient liquid and salt admission joined with a decent harmony among exercise and rest.

Studies including fasting regimens in individuals of underneath ordinary body weight, breastfeeding or pregnant ladies, youngsters, and the old have been generally scant; in these individuals, intermittent fasting ought to be started carefully, or not in the slightest degree. People exceptionally defenseless to hunger are not reasonable for a intermittent fasting routine, incorporating those with a neurological sickness; for instance, intermittent fasting is contraindicated in specific individuals with PD or AD who might be malnourished. Despite the fact that the part of intermittent fasting in intense contaminations has not been completely explained in people, intermittent fasting might be unfavorable in viral diseases (alternately, it very well might be defensive in bacterial diseases). Intermittent Fasting can in any case be considered in people with type 1 or 2 diabetes, gastro esophageal reflux, renal stones, and gout; in any case, it is shrewd to initially counsel a doctor experienced in intermittent fasting. Given the proof that fasting can improve or switch insulin obstruction, individuals with type 2 diabetes are generally ideal applicants.

Additionally, the danger of intermittent fasting-prompted hypoglycemia in type 2 diabetes is low; a new report looking at the impacts of type 2 diabetics clinging to a two-days-out of each week intermittent fasting routine more than 12 weeks exhibited that most members didn't encounter hypoglycemia, and no member experienced extreme hypoglycemia (characterized as an occasion needing the help of someone else for its amendment).

Common Adverse Effects

In a new, complete examination of 768 visits including people kept up on a therapeutically managed, water-just quick for at least two days, most antagonistic impacts were gentle to-direct and remembered (in plummeting request) weakness, sleep deprivation, sickness, migraine, hypertension (considered accidental, given that 97% of individuals with hypertension as an "unfavorable impact" likewise had hypertension as their prevailing clinical objection), presyncope, dyspepsia, back agony, and torment in a limit. It has for quite some time been realized that the underlying days of a period intermittent fasting are related with a characteristic diuresis, or "natriuresis of intermittent fasting," in which a lot of water and sodium are lost in the pee. In intermittent fasting periods enduring 24–48 hours or more, the natriuretic opens a person to drying out and low sodium levels, which whenever left untreated, can create manifestations like weakness, cerebral pain, and presyncope; much of the time, side effects identified with the natriuretic can be tried not to by guarantee satisfactory water and salt admission.

Rare Adverse Effects

Very uncommon unfriendly impacts have been archived in people going through delayed diets, including edema, serious hypokalemia, gut hindrance, urate nephrolithiasis, ventricular arrhythmias, and even demise; nonetheless, it is fundamental to perceive that these antagonistic occasions have happened in individuals going through incredibly drawn out intermittent fasting periods, many enduring a little while or months in length. Interestingly, out of 768 visits including people going through water-just intermittent fasting for at least two days, none of these uncommon antagonistic impacts happened.

2.11 Misconceptions of Intermittent Fasting

Now and again, disarray emerges with respect to the possible impacts of intermittent fasting in people. Normally, a comprehension of physiological setting permits any misinterpretations to be explained.

Symptomatic and Metabolic Effects of Intermittent Fasting

It is critical to separate the suggestive and metabolic impacts of a virtual end of calories (intermittent fasting) from those related with a serious, 40%–half calorie limitation. People going through momentary diets as often as possible report an absence of craving, which might be relative to the degree of ketosis accomplished, just as enhancements in energy, disposition, fearlessness, and personal satisfaction. Conversely, serious calorie limitation is related with determined appetite, weakness, peevishness, aloofness, and loss of sex drive. These differentiating suggestive impacts may result from recorded contrasts between serious calorie limitation and intermittent fasting regarding their consequences for the resting metabolic rate. The human body adjusts to a constant 20%–40% decrease in calorie consumption by bringing its resting metabolic rate down to generally a similar degree. Conversely, intermittent fasting invigorates a 5%–15% expansion in the resting metabolic rate, which by and large pinnacles a few days after the commencement of the intermittent fasting time frame, after which the metabolic rate brings down to pretty much its unique rate. The basic instruments for these differentiating metabolic reactions are to a great extent clarified by the way that calorie limitation diminishes by and large thoughtful action, while intermittent fasting builds it through the initiation of "counter-administrative" chemicals like GH, cortisol, and catecholamine.

Muscle Mass and Exercise Tolerance during Intermittent Fasting

The impacts of intermittent fasting on bulk and exercise resistance are as often as possible discussed. In any individual, the level of weight reduction, including muscle misfortune, relies upon their underlying muscle to fat ratio, calorie and protein admission, and exercise levels. In overweight and large people, protein admissions of 0.8–1.2 g per kg of body weight each day have a saving impact on slender mass. In any case, low and typical weight people show higher paces of protein oxidation comparative with energy consumption contrasted with hefty people, recommending that more slender individuals may require more protein per kg of body weight to keep up bulk.

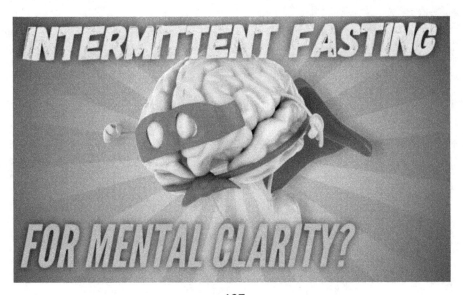

Notwithstanding sufficient protein consumption, ordinary exercise has additionally been appeared to forestall muscle misfortune in fat and typical weight people going through intermittent fasting regimens. In a 12-week study including stout people, consolidating ADF with perseverance practice three times each week decreased fat mass and held lean mass in a better way than either ADF or exercise alone. Additionally, two late examinations including solid youngsters showed that TRF joined with opposition practice three times each week brought about diminished fat mass and energy admission, though lean mass and strength were held. These discoveries propose that activity isn't essentially restricted by intermittent fasting; also, practicing in the abstained state may really be an ideal technique for diminishing fat mass while holding muscle.

Intermittent Fasting-Induced Insulin Resistance

It has for quite some time been perceived that intermittent fasting periods surpassing 48 hours in people are regularly joined by a reduction in skeletal muscle insulin affectability. This intermittent fasting-instigated insulin opposition, otherwise called "starvation diabetes," creates in the setting of hypoglycemia and hypoinsulinemia and presumably serves to restrict glucose take-up by skeletal muscle, guaranteeing that a consistent glucose supply consistently stays accessible for the compulsory necessities of the cerebrum. Consequently, intermittent fasting-instigated insulin opposition addresses an ordinary physiological transformation that plans to safeguard mind work. It is imperative to recognize intermittent fasting-instigated insulin obstruction from insulin opposition that creates in the setting of hyperglycemia and hyperinsulinemia, since the last is neurotic and may prompt sort 2 diabetes.

Compensatory Overeating During Intermittent Fasting

A last concern is that toward the finish of each intermittent fasting period, people may get defenseless to compensatory gorging, an impact that would moderate the useful impacts of the quick. For longer than a century, expanded yearning prompting "post-limitation hyperphagia" has been archived in individuals exposed to serious calorie limitation regimens. Conversely, late investigations of individuals on intermittent fasting regimens have not shown compensatory indulging on taking care of days. In addition, in investigations that have detailed an expansion in calorie admission on the taking care of days, the additional admission has still not made up for the general calorie deficiency prompted by the intermittent fasting time frames.

Evidence suggesting that Intermittent Fasting have improved Cognitive function

Possibly you skirt a feast to a great extent to attempt to get fit, or maybe you swear off eating in recognition of a strict occasion. In any case, what befalls your cerebrum when you do without food? Imprint Mattson, a neuroscientist at the National Institute on Aging and an educator at Johns Hopkins University, uncovers the amazing mind advantages of intermittent fasting.

The path we as researchers who study intermittent fasting characterize it isn't burning-through nourishment for a long sufficient timeframe to hoist the degrees of mixtures called ketones. In the fed express that is, the point at which you're not intermittent fasting glucose is the essential fuel utilized by cells, including neurons. Intermittent fasting drains the liver's store of glucose, inciting fat cells to deliver fats. The fats travel to the liver where they're changed over into ketones, which are basically little bits of fats that phones can use as a fuel source.

This metabolic switch going from utilizing glucose to utilizing ketones as a fuel source occurs after around 10 to 14 hours of not devouring food, contingent upon how dynamic you are. Exercise will speed up the beginning of the switch.

There are various kinds of intermittent fasting regimens. In lab creatures, the fundamental routine we use is substitute day intermittent fasting where the rodents or mice have no nourishment for a 24-hour time span, trailed by a 24-hour duration where they can eat, etc. Then again, you can confine the measure of time creatures approach food to a four-to six-hour window so that they're intermittent fasting somewhere in the range of 18 and 20 hours every day. In individuals, we've examined an intermittent fasting routine called the 5:2 eating regimen, where individuals eat regularly for five days out of the week and afterward eat just around 500 calories on the other two days.

In a creature in the wild, similar to a cougar or a wolf that hasn't killed any prey a long time, during that time they're practically running on ketones as opposed to glucose. Clearly, it's significant that their mind and body can work well in that abstained state. Furthermore, that is the thing that we're finding in lab creatures the cerebrum and body really perform better during intermittent fasting. On account of the mind, intellectual capacity, learning, memory, and sharpness are completely expanded by intermittent fasting. What's more, in the body, we as of late found that mice kept up on a substitute day intermittent fasting diet during a month of treadmill preparing have preferable perseverance over mice took care of consistently. So intermittent fasting upgraded the mice's actual presentation.

In lab creatures, intermittent fasting, just as exercise, invigorates the creation of a protein in nerve cells called cerebrum inferred neurotrophic factor, or BDNF. This protein assumes basic parts in learning, memory, and the age of new nerve cells in the hippocampus. BDNF likewise makes neurons more impervious to stretch. Intermittent fasting likewise triggers an interaction called autophagy, where cells eliminate harmed particles and useless mitochondria, and turns off cell development. So neurons are in a sort of "asset protection and stress obstruction" mode during intermittent fasting. At the point when the creature, and by extrapolation presumably the human, eats after intermittent fasting, neurons shift to a "development" mode they make heaps of proteins, develop, and structure new neurotransmitters. We think these patterns of metabolic test, regardless of whether its activity or intermittent fasting, and afterward a recuperation period may improve neuroplasticity, learning, memory, and the obstruction of the mind to pressure.

As of now, hardly any examinations have researched the intellectual advantages of intermittent fasting in people. We're in an investigation at the National Institute on Aging where we're taking individuals who are in danger of psychological hindrance as a result of their age and weight and haphazardly doling out them to either a 5:2 intermittent fasting diet or a control diet which is only guidance for smart dieting. Prior to beginning the eating regimen and afterward two months after the fact we're doing a battery of psychological tests with an attention on different parts of learning and memory. We're partially through the examination currently, however it will be for a little while before the end-product.

Conclusion

This audit gives proof to potential advantages of intermittent fasting, like decreased insulin, expanded IGF, improved metabolic guideline, expanded autophagy, diminished neuroinflammation, expanded degrees of BDNF, and improved conduct. The central issue is the impact of modifiable way of life factors in solid maturing. Numerous other way of life factors, like eating regimen, exercise, perception, and social advancement, have additionally been ensnared in life span, sound cerebrum maturing, and anticipation/treatment of neurodegenerative infections.

In a period of rising medical care costs and an expanding pervasiveness of neurological sickness, the presentation of a self-enabling, without cost, successful remedial choice for a scope of neurological issues would be a welcome expansion to the armamentarium of doctors. The present most basic neurological problems are in a general sense described by blemished digestion, on numerous levels. Given that fasting is a straightforward, multi-focused on, and basically "metabolic" treatment with a sound history for treating an assortment of neurological infections in creatures, it holds guarantee as a treatment for practically equivalent to sicknesses in people.

CPSIA information can be obtained
at www.ICGtesting.com
Printed in the USA
BVHW091022120521
606756BV00022B/1389